Wake Up! You're Snoring…

Wake Up! You're Snoring…

A Guide to Diagnosis and Treatment

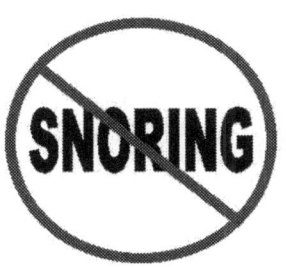

David O. Volpi, M.D.
Josh L. Werber, M.D.

http://www.wakeupyouresnoring.com

iUniverse, Inc.
New York Lincoln Shanghai

Wake Up! You're Snoring...
A Guide to Diagnosis and Treatment

iUniverse, Inc.

For information address:
iUniverse, Inc.
2021 Pine Lake Road, Suite 100
Lincoln, NE 68512
www.iuniverse.com

ISBN: 0-595-27031-X

Printed in the United States of America

To our wives and children

and to our parents

Contents

Introduction

As otolaryngologists, we see many patients who snore. Although many people are reluctant to admit they have a problem, it is thought that more than forty million Americans snore every night. People of all ages suffer from snoring, as you'll discover in the case studies we've presented in this book. We hope these stories will help you evaluate your snoring and help you make decisions about how or when to seek help.

The loss of sleep associated with snoring may be related to a serious medical condition called sleep apnea. Affecting one in ten middle-aged men and slightly fewer women, sleep apnea causes a victim's breathing to stop for more than ten seconds at a time—several times an hour. This particular sleep disorder puts people at risk for stroke, high blood pressure, and irregular heart rhythms.

Today's health consumers have a wide range of options and a greater freedom to choose treatment options than they have had at any time in history. This book will not only help you understand snoring, it will also provide you with information about nonsurgical and surgical treatments available to cure your snoring.

HOW TO USE THIS BOOK

The first few chapters in this book are designed to help you become acquainted with why people snore as well as the consequences of snoring. Because excess weight leads to difficulties with snoring, we have included chapters on weight management and exercise.

Subsequent chapters cover sleep apnea, treatment for snoring and sleep apnea, and resources for people who snore. Included in the resources chapter is a list of sleep support groups, sleep organizations in the United States and Europe, universities with programs in sleep medicine, board-certified sleep specialists, and accredited sleep centers around the country. Most of these listings include an e-mail and Web site address that you may use on the Internet.

1

Snore Wars

Although snoring might seem to be a very private habit, the consequences of snoring can upset relationships at work and at home. Most people ignore a snoring problem. They will often hide it and pretend that it doesn't exist. Acknowledging snoring is a responsible choice, and taking steps toward finding a solution can be very liberating. Although light snoring may have few consequences, heavy snoring carries great risk.

This chapter covers the consequences of snoring, including productivity due to daytime sleepiness and the burden snoring places on people who share a bedroom or physically occupy a bed near a loud snorer.

DAYTIME CONSEQUENCES OF SNORING

People who are sleep deprived are often irritable; they lack ability to concentrate, and overall productivity is limited because reaction time is slow and thinking becomes dull.

Because snorers are asleep while they snore, they're usually unaware of their problem. It may also be difficult for them to make a connection between snoring and daytime symptoms. Severe symptoms typically present in people who have sleep apnea include the following:

Morning Headaches

People with sleep apnea often suffer from morning headaches associated with a lack of oxygen during sleep.

Did You Know…
Sleep apnea has been found in 25–50% of people who have high blood pressure.

Irritability and a Feeling of Burnout

Sleep loss can build up over time. Chronic sleep deprivation can cause anxiety, erratic behavior, and agitation. Sleep researchers who have studied sleep deprivation have noticed aggressive behavior in people who are sleep deprived.

Poor Memory and Concentration Skills

Frequent awakenings associated with snoring and sleep apnea frequently cause problems with memory and concentration. People with this symptom may have difficulty with numbers; they may forget names and have problems with short and long-term memory.

Did You Know…
There are two kinds of sleep:

1. REM sleep, short for Rapid Eye Movement sleep, is a stage characterized by dreaming and rapid eye movement beneath closed eyelids. REM sleep occurs approximately every 90 minutes and lasts 5–30 minutes.

2. Delta sleep, or deep sleep, is called Non-REM sleep or NREM sleep. This type of sleep is associated with physical recovery and restoration. Those who are deprived of delta

Sleep Debt

Sleep debt is an ongoing need for sleep that accumulates and is carried into the daytime. As sleep debt builds up, there is an increased need to fall asleep during normal daytime activities. Frequently, people suffering from sleep debt will fall asleep whenever they're stationary. They'll doze off while they're reading, watching TV, sitting at a table or desk, or even driving. Sleep debt is also called ESD or Excessive Daytime Sleepiness.

Dry Mouth

A dry mouth in the morning is the result of sleeping with the mouth open. An obstruction in the nasal passageways is usually the cause. Sleeping with the mouth open leads to relaxation in the jaw muscles, which can lead to sleep apnea.

Depression

Frequent crying, early morning awakenings, a poor appetite, difficulty accomplishing routine tasks, and feelings of sadness are characteristics of depression that may be associated with a sleep problem.

Did You Know...
The most popular earplugs are made of wax or ear-contouring foam.

Poor Job Performance

People with sleep deprivation that results from snoring or sleep apnea are often so tired when they wake up, getting to work on time becomes a difficult challenge. Factors such as memory loss and poor concentration make tasks at work so difficult, a person's performance at work may become compromised, leading to poor quality work.

STRAINED RELATIONSHIPS

Snoring often places a difficult burden on partners, children, roommates, dorm members, and people who share sleeping accommodations on business or pleasure trips.

Depending on the severity, relatives and friends may grow resentful because of their own lost sleep. It is estimated that disruptive snorers can cause their partners to lose up to an hour's sleep per night. In 2001, the American College of Oral and Maxillofacial Surgeons studied 4,900 snoring couples and reported that 80 percent end up in separate bedrooms. In December 2001, ABC News reported that Albany, New York, apartment dweller Bruce Menia was asked to leave his home because his snoring was so loud.

Did You Know...
Hyperactive children and children with Attention Deficit Disorder may have a sleep disorder. Poor behavior and concentration at school are common signs of sleep apnea.

Case Study: Michelle
Michelle, a Manhattan real estate agent, describes her snoring as "louder than any man I have ever known." She admits her snores were so loud, friends would mock her and her boyfriends would disappear. At 39, she was convinced her snoring was the reason she was single.

Michelle's Somnoplasty
Michelle sought help for her snoring just as somnoplasty was introduced as a corrective procedure for snoring. In 2001, Michelle became one of the first New Yorkers to have a somnoplasty.

Somnoplasty is a nonsurgical medical procedure that uses radio-frequency to shrink the tissues in the roof of the mouth. It operates in the radio-frequency part of the electromagnetic spectrum at 465 Hz (pulses per second). The uvula and the soft palate can obstruct the upper airways, and somnoplasty uses heat to shrink their tissues. Although somnoplasty usually involves a single treatment, Michelle required two. The procedure is done under local anesthesia while a needle-like device is used to administer heat to the roof of the mouth.

Sorbet and Jell-O for Two Days
Somnoplasty procedures last about twenty minutes and Michelle reports, "There was no pain—just a little discomfort." Although she ate sorbet and Jell-O for two days, normal eating habits are not restricted after treatment. Most patients report mild swelling, a slight amount of speech distortion, and discomfort that typically lasts one to two days. Two months after her somnoplasty, Michelle met the love of her life, and her snoring is no longer a problem.

SNORING ETIQUETTE

If you have a problem with snoring and you're planning to spend one or more nights with colleagues, you may want to consider these suggestions:

Warn Your Colleagues You Snore

Before you make your hotel reservations for a business trip or leave for an overnight stay on a hiking or camping trip, speak up and warn your fellow travelers that you snore. Discussing your snoring in advance will help to avoid stress in your relationships.

Provide Earplugs

The person who snores should provide fellow travelers with earplugs.

Mask Your Snores

Sometimes snoring can be masked with the noise from a fan, a white noise CD, or a sound machine.

Travel with a Blow-Up Mattress

A blow-up mattress is a compact solution that can turn any separate room into a bedroom.

Did You Know…
In *Sleepless in Seattle*, Meg Ryan decides she cannot marry her boyfriend because he snores.

2

Why Do People Snore?

What structures in the nose and throat cause people to snore? Anatomically, even though we all have the same components in the nose and throat, there are large variations in the head and neck.

Weight can make a difference, injuries in the nose and throat can cause blockages in the airways, and some people are born with narrow passages.

To understand why people snore, it's helpful to review the route that air travels when we breathe and to understand what might potentially block the inflow of air while we sleep.

AIRWAYS IN THE NOSE

The structures inside the nose that may block breathing include the following (see figure 1):

Deviated Nasal Septum

A nasal septum consists of bone and cartilage, and its function is to separate the nasal cavity into right and left partitions. A nasal septum may take on an abnormal shape from a birth defect or when the nose is broken. A deviated nasal septum is one that has an uneven shape that may block breathing.

Nasal Polyps

A polyp is a small benign tumor that grows inside the nose or sinus cavity. One or more polyps may block breathing through the nose.

Nasal Turbinates

Nasal turbinates are bulky structures inside the nasal cavity made of ridge-shaped cartilage or soft bony tissue. They are covered by mucous membranes that clean, moisten, and warm inspired air.

Did You Know...
Doctors believe most people who have sleep apnea have never been diagnosed.

[figure 1]

Lateral wall of nose

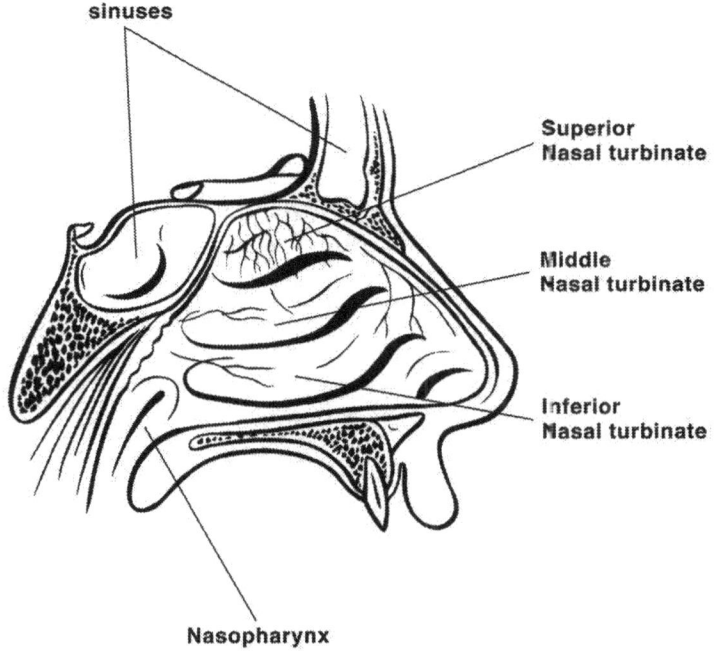

sinuses

Superior
Nasal turbinate

Middle
Nasal turbinate

Inferior
Nasal turbinate

Nasopharynx

AIRWAYS BETWEEN THE NOSE AND THROAT

The structures that lie between the nose and throat include the following (see figure 2):

Nasopharynx

This is the airway that connects the nasal passages to the throat. It includes the adenoids, which when enlarged, can cause nasal obstruction and snoring.

Sinuses

Sinuses are air-filled, mucosal-lined cavities located in the facial and cranial bones. Although their function is unknown, it is thought that they serve to decrease the weight of the skull or function as resonators for the voice.

Soft Palate

This soft tissue lies behind the roof of the mouth.

Did You Know…
Snoring is caused by mouth breathing. During sleep, the throat relaxes and the tongue falls into the airway in the back of the throat causing a vibration in the soft tissue.

AIRWAY IN THE THROAT

The structures inside the throat that may block breathing include the following (see figure 2):

Tongue

If the tongue is large and the musculature in the throat relaxes during sleep, the tongue may block the airway to the lungs.

Palate

The palate consists of two parts: a hard palate made of bone that extends between the teeth and a soft palate at the rear of the throat.

Uvula

The uvula is a soft fleshy bag that is located in the middle of the soft palate.

Tonsils

Located in the back of the mouth, one on each side, tonsils are mostly composed of lymphoid tissue that is involved in antibody production. Although antibody production is considered to be a good thing, it is thought that when the tonsils and/or the adenoids become dysfunctional, they become more of a liability than an asset. Like adenoids, tonsils may contribute to snoring and sleep apnea when they become enlarged.

Epiglottis

A flap of cartilage at the back of the tongue that closes off the windpipe when swallowing.

Larynx

Anatomical name for the voice box.

[figure 2]

Nose and Throat Anatomy

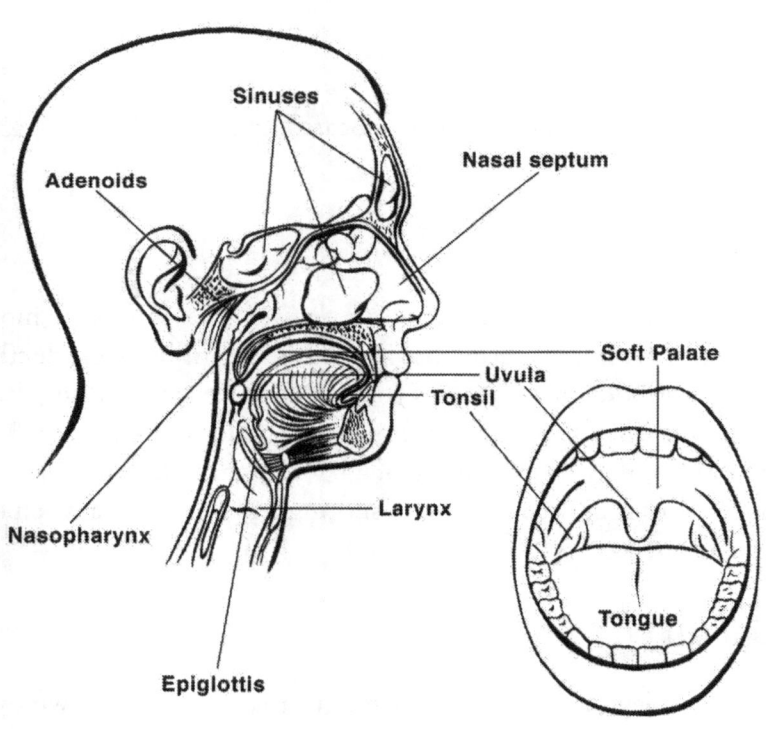

Did You Know...

Noise levels are measured in decibels (dB), and the loudest recorded snore measured 87 decibels. Noise over 30 decibels can disturb sleep. Here is a list of everyday sounds in decibels:

Whisper	30 dB
Human Voice	40 dB
Snoring	80 dB
Jackhammer	130 dB
Jet Plane Takeoff	120 dB
Vacuum Cleaner	70 dB

3

Understanding Your Snoring

If your snoring is related to a habit that is within your control, you may be able to solve your problem yourself. However, if your snoring is severe, you may need professional help to evaluate what may be a life-threatening disorder.

This chapter will guide you through the characteristics of snoring, provide you with information about lifestyle factors that may resolve your problem, and help you evaluate whether to seek the help of a physician.

FACTORS THAT CAUSE ADULTS TO SNORE

In the last thirty years, scientists have identified many factors that cause people to snore. Although factors such as gender, age, and abnormalities in the throat are impossible to control, for people who have mild or intermittent snoring, there are numerous variables that may be altered to try to solve a snoring problem. Your doctor can also help with your detective work at any time along the way.

Gender

Although scientists are not sure why, men are more likely to snore than women. Of those who snore, 50 percent are men and only 30 percent are women, although these percentages even out after menopause.

Men also snore louder than women. Loud snoring may be a sign of sleep apnea, a serious sleep disorder that causes breathing to stop for ten seconds or more periodically throughout the night.

Did You Know...
Sleep deprivation is a leading cause of accidents.

More men than women have sleep apnea. Studies show that the incidence of sleep apnea in men is approximately 9 percent and 4 percent in women.

Age

Snoring tends to be a condition that is more common in adults over 40 years of age. Body weight often increases with age, and an associated loss of muscle tone in soft neck tissue results in a constriction in the throat and neck air passageways.

Weight

What you eat and how much you eat will have an effect on your weight and the quality of your sleep. Typically, people who are obese have the most problems with respiratory symptoms during sleep.

Weight reduction should be one of the chief goals of the heavy person who snores. Typically, loss of a few pounds often reduces snoring.

Chin folds and a very large neck are physical characteristics that are linked to difficulties with snoring. Fatty tissue in the throat vibrates as a person sleeps, contributing to the snoring sound. Excess weight at any age leads to extra throat tissue that may block airways.

Did You Know…
Curly, the funniest of the Three Stooges, played the part of a sleeping train passenger with a clothespin on his nose in a 1947 film called *Hold That Lion*. When Moe would remove the clothespin, Curly would start snoring.

Geography/Location

People who live in cities report more difficulties with sleep than those who live in rural areas. Studies have shown that air pollution in cities has more serious health effects, including asthma, coughing, and snoring.

Body Position While Sleeping

When a person sleeps on his/her stomach or side, there is less snoring. It is thought that this may be because gravity causes the tongue to fall backward into the throat when the sleeper lies on his or her back.

Anatomic Abnormalities

Snoring may be caused by deformities such as a soft palate that is stiffer or longer than normal, a long uvula, a deviated septum, or enlarged tonsils and/or adenoids.

Genetics

Genes plays an indirect role in snoring. Because children with overweight parents are more likely to be overweight, they are also likely to snore. Snoring and sleep apnea are both associated with obesity.

Race/Ethnicity

Studies have shown that sleep apnea is more frequent in African-Americans than in Caucasians or Hispanics.

> **Did You Know...**
> When Robert Redford first encounters Paul Newman in *Butch Cassidy and the Sundance Kid*, Newman is asleep and snoring on the floor next to his bed.

Exercise

Regular activity and exercise lead to toned muscles that minimize snoring. Exercise helps us to maintain a healthy weight, a long life span, and optimal health.

Alcohol

Because alcohol relaxes muscles in the throat and upper air passageways, a drink in the evening may aggravate snoring. Although a drink at dinner will probably not affect the intermittent snorer, a person with sleep apnea should avoid alcohol at the end of the day.

> **Did You Know...**
> In Massachusetts, there's a law that says snoring is prohibited unless all bedroom windows are closed and securely locked.

Nicotine

Over time, smoking irritates the tissue in the air passageways, which causes swelling and results in breathing abnormalities. There is a strong correlation between smoking and snoring.

Drugs

Several medications have side effects that can cause snoring. Examples include the following:

Medications That Relax Air Passageways

Tranquilizers, sleeping pills and antihistamines relax the muscles in the throat and upper air passageways that lead to snoring.

Pain Medication (Particularly Narcotics)

A drug that causes sedation can cause snoring.

Oral Contraceptives and Estrogens

Oral contraceptives and estrogens can cause hormonal changes that affect the upper airway passages.

High Blood Pressure Medication

Hypothyroidism

Thyroid deficiency, or hypothyroidism, causes excessive daytime sleepiness and snoring that is similar to sleep apnea. If you snore, you may want to ask your doctor for a thyroid function test to rule out hypothyroidism.

Did You Know…
If you need an alarm clock to wake up every morning, you may be sleep deprived.

Environmental Factors

Numerous environmental factors may cause snoring. Examples include the following:

Allergens. Common allergens such as pollen, dust, dust mites, and animal hair can cause irritation or swelling in the nose and throat. Such allergic reactions can lead to snoring.

Air Pollutants. Chemicals, sprays, fumes, and smoke are common irritating substances that can irritate air passageways and obstruct breathing.

Humidity. If the air in your home is very dry, your nose may become stuffed up, causing mouth breathing and snoring.

FACTORS THAT CAUSE CHILDREN TO SNORE

Children, teens, and young adults are subject to many of the same snore-related factors as adults, with the following distinctions:

Gender

In young adults, males are ten times more likely to snore than females.

Sleep apnea in children is equally distributed among males and females.

Did You Know...
Apnea is a Greek word that means without breath. Apnea is characterized by loud snoring and periods of holding the breath.

Tonsillitis or Enlarged Adenoids

In children, enlarged tonsils or adenoids frequently cause blockage that can cause snoring. Because tonsils and adenoids begin to shrink as children reach early adolescence, snoring may become less of a problem.

Weight

Obesity is a common factor in sleep apnea regardless of a person's age. Of American children, 10 percent are obese and 25 percent of the child population is overweight.

ARE YOU OVERWEIGHT?

Body Mass Index (BMI) is considered to be an accurate measure of body fat, and a BMI greater than 28 is considered to be in the obese range. While 60 percent of American adults are considered overweight, 27 percent of these are considered to be obese.

A BMI of 19 to 25 is considered to be a healthy weight, and a BMI under 19 is considered to be underweight.

To calculate your BMI:

    a.   Multiply body weight in pounds by 700.

    b.   Divide this number by height in inches.

    c.   Divide this number by height (in inches) again.

Example:
Mary Lou weighs 200 pounds and she is 5 feet 8 inches tall. To calculate her BMI:

    a.   200 x 700=140,000

    b.   140,000/68=2058.82

    c.   2058.82/68=30.27

With a BMI of 30.27, Mary Lou would be considered obese.

Did You Know...
Swollen tonsils can block a child's air passageways and cause snoring.

TRACK YOUR SNORING WITH A SLEEP DIARY

The idea of keeping a sleep diary to track your snoring may appeal to some, but to others the idea may seem like a nuisance. If your snoring is keeping your partner awake, perhaps he/she can help you with your diary or provide the necessary motivation you may need to get started.

A sleep diary will help you track how you feel after a night's sleep; the medications you take on a daily basis, as well as smoking, eating, and exercise. Light or intermittent snoring can often be solved with adjustments in habits that have become part of your lifestyle.

Either enlarge the following chart with a photocopier or use the charts as a guide to create your own. You'll need to keep your sleep diary near your bed. You might consider taping it to a wall or closet door so you don't forget to add important details on a daily basis. Fill out the sleep diary each morning and evening.

[figure 3]

Sleep Diary	Sun A.M.	Sun P.M.	Mon A.M.	Mon P.M.	Tue P.M.	Tue A.M.	Tue P.M.	Wed A.M.	Wed P.M.	Thur A.M.	Thur P.M.	Fri A.M.	Fri P.M.	Sat A.M.	Sat. P.M.
Date															
Morning questions															
Did you snore last night? (Use the Mayo Clinic grade described at the end of this chapter.)															
Did you take any medications before bed?															
Did you have alcohol 4 hours before bed?															
How many hours did you sleep?															
How well did you sleep? (use a 1-to-10 scale)															
Evening questions															
Did you feel sleepy today?															
Did you smoke today?															
Did you exercise today?															

Example:

George is a smoker who would like to track the relationship between his smoking and snoring. To get started with his sleep diary, George takes the sleep diary to Kinko's and uses a photocopier to scale the chart to 165 percent.

Starting on a Sunday night, George records the date at the top of the column labeled Sun p.m. and writes Yes next to the question Did you smoke today?

The next morning, George's wife, Cynthia, helps him grade his snores using the Mayo Clinic's Grades (see a description of the Mayo Clinic's Grades at the end of this chapter). Cynthia decides to give George's snores a Grade 3, so he adds a 3 in the Mon. A.M. box next to the question Did you snore last night?

ADDING YOUR OWN VARIABLES TO THE DIARY

You may want to add additional variables to your sleep diary. Add rows to your diary and conduct experiments by recording data on a daily basis. Examples include the following:

- You may suspect a feather pillow has been causing an allergic reaction.
- The quality of the air in your bedroom may be altered with an air filter.
- Regular changes in heating and air conditioning filters may control dust in the home.
- Wall-to-wall carpeting may contain allergens such as dust and formaldehyde.
- A 30–40 percent humidity level is an ideal level for any room in the home. The humidity in your bedroom may be altered with a humidifier if the air is excessively dry. (Note: Humidity levels should not be too high because humidity over 45 percent creates a favorable breeding environment for dust mites that are a common allergen in the bedroom. If a humidifier is used, it should be cleaned regularly to prevent mold growth.)
- A potential dust mite problem in the bedroom may be solved by washing bedding each week in water above 130 degrees and using allergen-proof covers for the mattress and pillows.
- Small soft furnishings such as toys and scatter cushions may contain a dust mite colony that can be eliminated at a high temperature in a dryer.
- When you're away from home, record details about your snores, for example, while you're on vacation.

Example:

Donald is a nonsmoker who is not overweight, but he has a lifelong history of allergies. His wife has been complaining about his snoring and he's decided to use a sleep diary to track the relationship between his snoring and possible environmental factors in their bedroom.

As George did, Donald takes the sleep diary to Kinko's and uses a photocopier to scale the chart to 165 percent.

Donald suspects that his home's forced-air heating system may be drying out the air in his home and causing his nasal passageways to be dry and irritated. Using the extra rows provided on the chart, Donald writes Humidifier (Yes/No) on an empty line and runs the humidifier in his bedroom for a few hours each day for several days. Starting on a Sunday night, Donald records the date at the top of the column labeled Sun P.M. and writes Yes in the line labeled Humidifier (Yes/No).

The next morning, Donald's wife, Susan, helps him grade his snores using the Mayo Clinic's Grades (see a description of the Mayo Clinic's Grades at the end of this chapter). Susan decides to give Donald's snores a Grade 2, so he adds a 2 in the Mon A.M. box next to the question Did you snore last night? Although Donald's snores have not stopped, Susan feels the humidifier has a positive effect on Donald's snoring. Because of Donald's history of allergies, they decide to continue to use the sleep diary to investigate other variables in their bedroom, including an air filter, an alternate pillow, and a bedroom rug.

EVALUATING ENTRIES IN YOUR SLEEP DIARY

The purpose of the sleep diary is to narrow down the variables that may be causing you to snore. You'll need to record data for at least a week or possibly two to three weeks. Some people who create a sleep diary will stumble on a solution themselves, but others will discover they need the help of a professional.

> **Did You Know...**
> Foods that contain the amino acid tyramine will keep you awake. Examples include cheese, sugar, ham, bacon, and tomatoes.

WHEN TO CONSULT A DOCTOR

If you snore, there is a chance you may also have sleep apnea, which can be a serious medical problem. If your snoring is very loud and you have excessive daytime sleepiness, you should consult a doctor.

Sleep loss impairs a person's ability to perform tasks involving memory, learning, reasoning, and mathematical processes.

Dr. Nelson B. Powell, a dentist and physician at Stanford University, recently led a research team that measured the response times of people who were sleep deprived. They recruited 113 patients with mild to moderate sleep apnea and compared their reaction times with 80 normal volunteers who had slept well for three consecutive nights.

The Stanford study showed severe impairment in people with only mild to moderate sleep disturbances. Results showed reaction times that were similar to people who were legally drunk. The results of the study were published in the October 1999 issue of *Laryngoscope* and suggest that risks of accidents due to sleepiness—especially in high risk occupations such as those of pilots, truck drivers, and train engineers are very high in the sleep deprived. The National Highway Traffic Safety Administration (NHTSA) already knows that insufficient sleep can be dangerous and lead to fatal automobile accidents. The NHTSA has estimated that more than two hundred thousand auto accidents a year are fatigue related.

The severity of the snoring is often an indicator of whether you have sleep apnea and need treatment.

It may be hard for you to assess the severity of your snores. If you live alone, you might consider taping your snores to determine if they're loud. A partner or family member will be able to tell you how loud or how frequently you snore.

The Mayo Clinic's Sleep Disorders Center grades snoring from a bed partner's point of view:

Grade 1: Heard only if you listen close to the face
Grade 2: Heard in the room
Grade 3: Heard just outside the bedroom with the door open
Grade 4: Heard outside the bedroom with the door closed

DIAGNOSTIC TESTS

Once you decide to seek the advice of a doctor, you may be guided through one or more of the following diagnostic tests:

Nose and Throat Examination

A nose and throat exam will most likely be a starting point that will reveal potential blockages such as nasal obstruction, a large uvula, enlarged tonsils, or an enlarged tongue. This short exam will help your doctor identify the possible abnormalities that may cause snoring.

X-ray or Computerized Tomography Scan (CT)

If your doctor needs a detailed image of your sinuses, he or she may order a CT scan. This test provides a detailed cross-sectional image of the sinuses and can be used to help identify the severity of infection inside the sinus cavities.

Allergy Tests

Identification of allergens that cause nasal congestion is a highly specific specialty that may involve skin or blood tests. In all likelihood, if your doctor feels you need allergy tests, he/she will refer you to an allergist for specialized testing.

Did You Know...
Foods that contain tryptophan promote sleep. Examples include milk, honey, egg whites, tuna, and turkey.

Case Study: Elana

When six-year-old Elana's parents first brought her to the office, she had a several-year history of loud snoring, mouth breathing and a nasal voice. Her symptoms were year-round but worse during the cold season. Elana also had difficulty swallowing and was a poor eater.

Elana's Enlarged Tonsils

During her physical exam, Elana appeared to be a thin girl with an open-mouth breathing pattern and hyponasal-sounding speech. A throat exam revealed enlarged tonsils that were touching each other in what is known as a "kissing pattern." Elana's parents described her as a restless sleeper. Although she frequently slept for eleven hours, she appeared to be tired. She had previously been diagnosed as "allergic" but found no relief from antihistamines or nasal steroid sprays. At the conclusion of her exam, Elana was diagnosed with adenotonsillar obstruction with related sleep disordered breathing. A tonsillectomy and adenoidectomy were both recommended. Elana's parents elected to schedule outpatient surgery the following month.

Snoring Stopped the Night of the Surgery

Ten days following her adenotonsillectomy, Elana's mother brought her to the office for a follow-up visit and reported that she had stopped snoring the night of the surgery. Although she had a painful sore throat for three days following the surgery, she was now eating normally and had returned to school.

A physical exam revealed Elana was breathing through her nose with her mouth closed. Her voice was no longer nasal but was somewhat high-pitched. Her parents were informed that a squeaky voice was common after a tonsillectomy and that her voice would return to normal in a few weeks. A throat exam revealed an open space with white patches, indicating that healing was taking place. Two months later, Elana's mother called to report that Elana had gained four pounds and seemed "more energetic."

4

Weight Management

Because weight is the most common cause of snoring, weight management is an important goal for patients who snore. Although obesity is preventable, there is no single solution to weight management. There are vast differences in the human metabolism just as there are differences in anatomy.

Even though many diet and exercise books promote a low-calorie solution for losing weight, the truth is that everyone's metabolism is unique and you'll need to explore what diet is right for you.

This chapter describes a range of popular diets by today's leading experts. A basic familiarity with what these experts have to say will get you started on the road to self-discovery. If you have a weight management problem, you'll need to do some reading and experiment with a few different approaches to dieting. You'll discover that your results will speak for themselves. In addition to an overview of what diet authorities have to say, we've also included an expert's tips on how to listen to your body when you're evaluating different diets.

YO-YO DIETING

The National Institutes of Health recently reported that over 97 million Americans are now obese or significantly overweight. Surprisingly, the incidence of obesity in the United States has actually increased by over 30 percent in the last fifteen years.

Even though Americans are more weight conscious than ever before, most people have a very hard time losing weight and keeping it off. This is because of a phenomenon known as the "yo-yo effect." In other words:

- People often manage to lose a significant amount of weight after they initiate a diet, but like a yo-yo, the excess weight frequently comes right back again.
- Over 90 percent of people who diet fail to achieve any significant degree of success over the long term. Many people try multiple weight loss approaches over a period of many years. As a result, their weight tends to go up and down over and over again.

Did You Know...
The *Guinness Book of World Records* lists Melvin Switzer of South Hampton, England, as the record holder for the loudest snore. His snores measured 91 decibels.

WEIGHT LOSS VS. WEIGHT NORMALIZATION

Many leading nutritional experts believe that chronic obesity is not an isolated physical problem. Rather, many professionals view it as a symptom of metabolic or physiological imbalances that need to be corrected with a holistic and long-term approach to eating well.

The reason that most diets fail is that many people try to "force" weight off the body in an unhealthy or unnatural way. In other words, they focus on dropping pounds or losing weight in a rapid fashion, as opposed to normalizing their weight in a more natural way over a longer period of time.

Here are some issues to consider:

- Health consumers often gravitate toward various kinds of crash diets that promise instant results. Many of these approaches are one-dimensional or artificial, that is, they may succeed in helping people drop weight quickly, but unless dieters can correct underlying metabolic imbalances, these methods are not likely to produce long-term results.
- Each year, Americans spend billions of dollars on weight-loss diets and packaged food products and all sorts of quick fix solutions such as liquid diet drinks, appetite suppressants, diuretics, and diet pills designed to speed up the metabolism.
- A far better solution is to focus on making intelligent food choices designed to build and maintain health, as opposed to the narrower goal of simply dropping pounds.
- When good health becomes the primary goal, people can take the time to identify diets that are satisfying and sustainable, and comprised of wholesome foods that work well to balance the body chemistry over the long haul.
- Being lean and fit is actually a by-product or side effect of good health.

YOUR METABOLISM IS UNIQUE

Metabolism is the sum of all the biochemical processes that are required to sustain human life. Examples of metabolic activities are digestion, respiration, circulation, growth and repair of body tissue, and reproductive functions. All of these metabolic activities require energy in the form of food and nutrients. That's why the food choices you make have such a powerful impact on your health and well-being.

Dietary Building Blocks

All human beings need a full spectrum of nutrients, including proteins, carbohydrates, and fats. These are known as macronutrients because they are the fundamental building blocks of any healthy diet.

Did You Know…
In *Ferris Bueller's Day Off*, Ferris rigs an audio tape of his snores to convince his parents that he's alseep in his room.

[figure 4]

Macronutrients

Protein

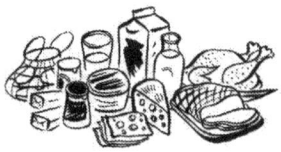

Sources: Protein sources include meat, poultry, and dairy products.

Functions: Proteins are used for building new cells that make up tissue, antibodies, enzymes, and blood cells.

Carbohydrate

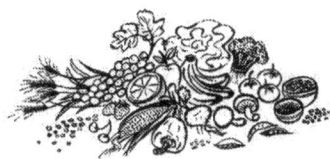

Sources: Carbohydrate sources are divided into complex carbohydrates or starches and simple carbohydrates or sugars. Comples sources include whole grains, vegetables, and fruits. Simple sources include honey, syrup candy, and most desserts.

Functions: Carbohydrates function as an energy source when they're broken down into glucose.

Fat

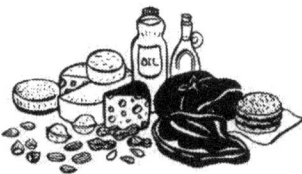

Sources: Fat sources include oils, nuts, meat, and cheese.

Functions: Fats protext the integrity of cell membranes and provide a source of stored energy. They play an important role in hormone synthesis, maintenance of the skin, and antiinflamatory processes.

The Importance of Omega-3 Fatty Acids

Researchers believe that approximately 60 percent of Americans are deficient in omega-3 fatty acids which play an important role in the prevention of coronary heart disease, hypertension, arthritis, and cancer. Omega-3 fatty acid, also known as linolenic acid, reduces serum triglyceride or the "hard" fat that cannot be used by the body.

Omega-3 and omega-6 fatty acids are polyunsaturated fats that are called essential because we need to obtain them from food. In contrast, non-essential amino acids are amino acids that your body can manufacture out of other chemicals found in your body. Although flax oil has become a popular source of omega-3 and omega-6 fatty acids, Udo Erasmus, author of *Fats That Heal Fats That Kill*, believes flax oil is too rich in omega-3 fatty acid compared to omega-6 (about four times as much omega-3 as omega-6). He explains that a blended oil with three times as much omega-3 as omega-6 provides the best balance for optimum health.

Oz Garcia, author of *The Healthy High Tech Body*, includes DHA, an omega-3 fatty acid, in his list of key nutrients. Found in fish and olive oils, DHA is an effective anti-inflammatory and may also increase neuronal fluidity.

Biochemical Individuality

Because of heredity or genetic differences between people, there is no single diet that works well for everyone. For instance, some people do well on diets comprised of larger amounts of protein and fat, but others do well on diets made up of larger amounts of carbohydrates. This is why some people can lose weight and feel energized and healthy on diets higher in heavier, fatty foods like meat and cheese, but others need large quantities of lighter foods like grains and vegetables in order to stay slim and healthy.

High Protein vs. Low Protein Diets

Currently there is a great deal of controversy among dietary experts about what constitutes a healthy diet. A national debate has emerged that focuses primarily on how much protein, carbohydrate, and fat people should consume. Popular nutritional experts such as Dr. Robert Atkins believe that high-protein diets are the only sensible approach to losing weight and avoiding chronic health problems. Other leading experts insist that just the opposite is true. They believe that low-protein diets can prevent health problems of all kinds, ranging from obesity to heart disease to chronic fatigue and diabetes.

Plant Protein vs. Animal Protein

In the last several decades, vegetarianism has become increasingly popular. Even fast food chains offer salads and veggie burgers.

Essential Amino Acids

Although some people thrive as vegetarians, many people who declare themselves vegetarians often do not understand the consequences of restricting their diet to plant protein. Animal protein contains twenty eight essential amino acids required to build important components in the body, such as blood cells, muscle tissue, and antibodies. Although it is possible to combine plant proteins to assemble these essential amino acids in vegetarian meals, it is very difficult.

Annemarie Colbin, a well-known proponent of vegetarianism and author of *The Natural Gourmet* and *Food and Healing*, admits that vegetarian meals are not for everyone.

Frank Ludde, a metabolic specialist in Vancouver, British Columbia, explains that adults need approximately fifty to sixty grams of usable protein per day to maintain the body's essential systems. Even though animal protein contains essential amino acids, Frank Ludde explains that the protein found in beef, chicken, and fish is not all usable by the human body. For example, a serving of one of these contains approximately 15 to 20 percent usable protein. Eggs, which also provide the body with all of the essential amino acids, contain

PERSONALIZED DIETARY SOLUTIONS

In recent years, many health experts and health consumers have come to the conclusion that no single diet works well for everyone. There is an increasing amount of evidence that suggests one-size-fits-all dietary solutions are not very effective. You may have noticed that the very same foods that leave one person feeling lethargic and hungry between meals may enable another person to feel energized and satisfied for hours at a time. You may be able to demonstrate this yourself by experimenting with different diets to see what foods and food combinations enable you to look and feel your best.

POPULAR DIETS BY LEADING EXPERTS

The following section includes a list of popular diet books that represent very different points of view with respect to the macronutrients. They range from high-protein diets to low-protein diets to something in between. Also included are a number of books that enable people to customize or personalize dietary solutions for themselves based on the unique aspects of their body chemistry.

Dr. Atkin's New Diet Revolution by Robert C. Atkins, M.D.

Dr. Atkins advocates a diet that is high in protein and very low in carbohydrates, which limits the body's production of insulin. Limited insulin production results in diminished food cravings and a reduction in fat storage in body tissues.

Similar books include *Protein Power* by Michael R. Eades, *The Carbohydrate Addict's Diet* by Rachael F. Heller, and *Sugar Busters!* by H. Leighton Steward.

High-protein diets are controversial because some health professionals consider them to be inappropriate and unbalanced solutions if they are adhered to for any length of time. On the other hand, some people seem to do very well by incorporating larger quantities of protein in their diets. In addition, after losing an initial amount of weight, dieters can always incorporate larger quantities of carbohydrates into their regimens until they achieve a balance that feels right for them.

Eat More, Weigh Less by Dean Ornish, M.D.

Like many other advocates of vegetarian-style meals, Dr. Ornish is a strong proponent of low-fat, low-protein, high-carbohydrate diets. He believes that excess dietary fat can interfere with healthy metabolic processes and should be heavily restricted in the daily diet. Dr. Ornish's studies have revealed that many people who follow his dietary advice have successfully lost weight, lowered their cholesterol, and reduced their chances for developing heart disease and other serious illnesses.

The Zone by Barry Sears, Ph.D.

As a former Massachusetts Institute of Technology, biochemical researcher, Dr. Sears is a proponent of 40-30-30 nutrition. He believes that people can lose weight and achieve multiple health benefits by eating just the right combination of macronutrients at each meal. Dr. Sears maintains that the ideal ration for each meal should be 40 percent high-fiber carbohydrate, 30 percent high-quality protein, and 30 percent fat. According to the author of this very popular dietary system, 40-30-30 meals create healthy hormonal responses that burn stored body fat while having a positive effect on many other bodily functions.

Other popular books on the topic of customized nutrition include:

- *Dr. Abravanel's Body Type Diet and Lifetime Nutrition Plan* by Elliot D. Abravanel.
- *Eat Right 4 Your Type* by Dr. Peter J. D'Adamo.

> **Did You Know...**
> Edible oils are vulnerable to light, heat, and oxygen. These elements can promote oxidation, causing an oil to turn rancid. Oils sold in tin cans are the most well protected.

LISTEN TO YOUR BODY

In the book *The Metabolic Typing Diet*, author/nutritionist William Linz Wolcott writes about the importance of finding a diet that is tailored to your own unique body chemistry. The book provides simple techniques readers can use to identify their "metabolic type," and in turn identify a specific combination of protein, fat, and carbohydrates that will meet their individual needs for these nutrients.

Many nutritional experts believe you can tell a great deal about what type of diet is right for you just by listening to your body. When you eat meals that suit your body chemistry, here are some of the positive reactions you should experience:

- You should feel full and free of hunger for four to five hours after eating.
- You should enjoy sustained physical and mental energy throughout the day.
- You should be free of food cravings for sweets and starchy foods.
- You should be free of common digestive problems such as indigestion and bloating.
- You should be free of fatigue, irritability, hyperactivity, and difficulty concentrating.
- You should have a general sense of well-being and a positive mental outlook.

Reversing Factors That Impede Progress

Moods can create obstacles and detract from the feelings of self-confidence that you'll need to make changes in your lifestyle. The following tips may help you combat negative feelings or moods:

Positive Self-Talk

The subconscious mind is very sensitive to negative thoughts. Self-talk, or stating positive intentions aloud, is a powerful way to program your mind for success. Creating movies in your mind is another way to program your subconscious. Football coaches use this technique with the athletes they train. Before a game, players often create "movies" in their minds and see themselves reaching their goals.

Create a Journal

Many people successfully purge negative thoughts by writing their feelings in a journal. If this technique works for you, create a journal and record your feelings each day. Look critically at whether your thoughts are sabotaging your ability to reach your goals.

Exercise

Exercise, particularly aerobic activities such as running, walking, and cycling, release endorphins in the brain that cause you to have feelings of well-being.

Eliminate Sugar from Your Diet

An addiction to sugar leads to irregularities in blood sugar levels that can lead to mood swings. When sugar is first absorbed into your bloodstream, you will experience a sugar high that will lead to a sugar low within a few hours.

Self-assessment: Common Challenges

Sometimes there are underlying factors that are related to the life-style issues that cause snoring. Examples include weight management and an addiction to alcohol:

Eating Disorders

1.   Do you have food cravings or go on food b nges?

2.   Do you eat when you're upset?

Addictions

1.   Are you addicted to cigarettes or caffeine?

2.   Do you drink too much?

Depression

1.   Have you experienced a change in your eating habits?

2.   Have there been changes in your sleep patterns or your ability to concentrate?

Relationships

1.   Is there an unhealthy pattern in any of your close personal relationships?

2.   Are you involved in an emotional or physically abusive relationship?

5

Exercise

Exercise is essential for maintaining a healthy weight. The first step is to identify a diet that's right for you, one comprised of wholesome foods and food combinations that will optimize your body's ability to repair, rebuild, and regulate itself. The second crucial step involved in achieving your ideal weight is to invest a little time and energy in exercises that you find enjoyable and compatible with your lifestyle.

BENEFITS OF AN ACTIVE LIFESTYLE

Rest assured that it is not necessary to join a health club or hire a personal trainer or tire yourself out with prolonged and difficult exercise routines.

There are plenty of exercises that are easy as well as enjoyable. It's important to pick simple exercise routines that you can look forward to, since consistency will yield tremendous benefits.

In addition to transforming your physical appearance, here are some of the benefits you can expect if you exercise on a regular basis:

- Stress reduction
- Diminished feelings of anxiety and depression
- Improved psychological well-being
- Enhanced self-image
- Improved quality of sleep

- Increased strength and endurance
- Enhanced youthfulness and vigor

TWO BASIC CATEGORIES OF EXERCISE

There are two basic types of exercise: aerobic and anaerobic. Aerobic exercises have the capacity to burn up lots of calories and fat, and in the process they use up plenty of oxygen.

Popular aerobic exercises include jogging, swimming, bicycling, tennis, roller blading, hiking, running on a treadmill, and working out on a stationery bike. These kinds of activities assist the body in achieving metabolic equilibrium. They also provide short-term benefits in terms of weight reduction.

Anaerobic exercises are very different. They do not use a great deal of oxygen, and they are not designed to burn up significant amounts of calories and fat. Weight lifting and resistance training, or strength training, are anaerobic activities designed to build strength and lean muscle tissue. This helps speed up the metabolic rate, and this in turn provides longer-term weight loss benefits.

THE IMPORTANCE OF STRENGTH TRAINING

The muscle that you build with strength training will consume calories and stored fat. In contrast, dieters who simply limit their calories will lose muscle. By combining strength training with a weight-reduction program, you will be able to maintain muscle while maintaining an ideal weight.

BIG MUSCLES VS. SMALL MUSCLES

There are over two hundered muscles in the human body that are organized into muscle groups. To plan an effective regimen, it is not important to choose exercises that work out every muscle in your body. Most trainers focus on muscle groups, and they recommend exercises that train the larger muscles for people who have limited time or who are not naturally drawn to exercise.

Anatomically, there are different-sized muscles in the body that may be categorized as big muscles and small muscles. Although these categories are loosely defined, most people would agree that the chest, back, and legs are considered to be the big muscles in the body.

[figure 5]

Muscles in the Human Body

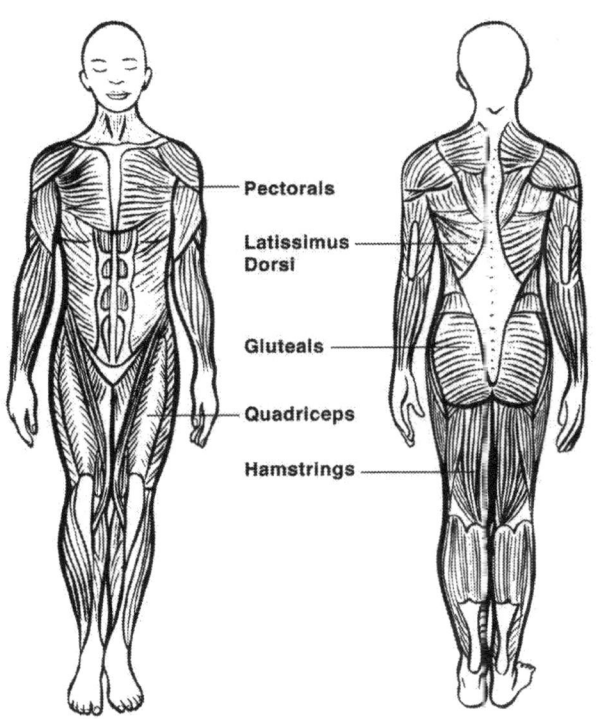

Pectorals

Latissimus Dorsi

Gluteals

Quadriceps

Hamstrings

Big Muscles in the Human Body

Muscle Location	Muscle Description
Chest	*Pectorals* Nicknamed pecs, the pectoral muscles consist of a large fan-shaped muscle located in the upper chest.
Back	*Latisimus dorsi* Nicknamed lats, the latisimus dorsi muscles are located across the middle of the back.
	Gluteals Nicknamed glutes, this group of muscles includes the gluteus maximus that covers the rear.
Legs	*Quadriceps* The quadriceps group of muscles make up the front of the thigh.
	Hamstrings The hamstring muscles make up the back of the thigh.

Too Busy to Join a Gym?

Although a gym can provide an ideal environment for an exercise program, many people who lead busy lives find it physically impossible to visit a gym on a regular basis.

Although it does require you to set aside some time, walking is an uncomplicated form of exercise that is easy and very accessible. Studies have shown that walking regularly is as effective as jogging in contributing to overall fitness.

The Inactive Person's Guide to Walking

Many people consider walking to be the perfect exercise. It is an exercise that does not require athletic ability, it is very low risk, and it does not put stress on the body. If you're not getting enough exerise, consider taking up walking, since brisk walks can burn up to three hundred calories per hour. Also consider the following tips:

Find Someone to Walk With
Sharing a nice long walk with a friend is a fun way to socialize.

Join a Walking or Hiking Club
If you have trouble finding someone to share a walk, consider joining a walking or hiking club.

Choose a Comfortable Pair of Shoes
Walking will require comfortable, supportive walking shoes. Try to find a waterproof pair so you won't be put off by walking in the rain, and look for cushioning if you plan to walk on concrete sidewalks. If you walk on natural paths, you may need a pair of light-weight hiking shoes. Many people who hike on trails also wear treaded trail sandals, which are cool in hot weather.

Dress for the Weather
Layered clothing is practical in hot weather or cold. Choose fabrics that are breathable, and take an umbrella if you think it might rain.

Plan Your Route
Your first concern when you plan your route should be safety. Plan a familiar route through major cross-streets and intersections that can help you get your bearings if you make a wrong turn. Look for points of interest such as parks, historic areas, or shopping districts. Many people like to combine errands with their walks.

Walking for Weight Control: How Long?
For weight loss, you will need to walk almost every day of the week. Take time off if you feel worn out, but try to start walking again as soon as possible.

Track Your Walks
A pedometer is a device that senses body motion and counts footsteps. The simplest pedometers count steps and display steps and/or distance. For weight loss, you should try to walk 4,000 to 6,000 steps each day.

For people who are schedule challenged, exercise workout at home may be a possible solution. Fitness trainers recommend Thera-Band Resistive Exercise Bands (www.thera-band.com) for people who wish to exercise at home and while traveling. These low-cost stretch bands provide a portable and lightweight means to perform resistive exercise at home or in a hotel room. Available in eight color-coded levels of resistance, the bands may be looped around stationary objects such as door knobs, or table legs. The exercise bands come with an illustrated brochure that contains suggested exercises that may be performed to strengthen the big muscle groups.

Thera-Band System of Progressive Resistance

Band Color	Description
Tan	Extra thin weight—provides the least resistance
Yellow	Thin weight
Red	Medium weight
Green	Heavy weight
Blue	Extra heavy weight
Black	Special heavy weight
Silver	Super heavy
Gold	Maximum resistance

Thera-Band Kits

Kit	Description
Light Pack	Contains a yellow, red, and green band (6 foot length)
Heavy Pack	Contains a green, blue, and black band (6 foot length)

6

Sleep Apnea

Sleep apnea is the most common sleep disorder, and it's also the most dangerous. People who suffer from sleep apnea stop breathing dozens of times during sleep and may not breathe for as much as three fourths of the time they're asleep.

The interval during sleep when breathing stops is called an apneic event. The word *apnea* comes from a Greek prefix *a*, meaning "no," and the Greek word *pnoia*, meaning "breath." The word *hypopnea* refers to less breathing. A hypopneic event occurs when the flow of air is reduced for ten seconds or more.

Apnea is particularly severe and life threatening when there are more than twenty or thirty events per hour. Because the heart is sensitive to oxygen levels in the blood, apnea is most dangerous in people with heart disease.

This chapter describes the types of sleep apnea, the serious side effects, and the methods currently used to diagnose the problem.

TYPES OF SLEEP APNEA

There are three types of sleep apnea, classified here according to their causes:

Obstructive Sleep Apnea (OSA)

As its name implies, obstructive sleep apnea is related to an obstructed upper airway, and it is the most common type as well as the most serious. Soft tissue in the palate, throat, or tongue may block the flow of air as a person struggles to breathe.

Characteristics of Obstructive Sleep Apnea

Characteristic	Description
Snoring	**Usually very loud**
Anatomical Abnormality	Narrow Pharynx (throat) Short, heavy neck Large tonsils Short lower jaw Large tongue Large Uvula Soft, fleshy palate Nasal congestion from allergies or deviated septum
Body Weight	Overweight people may have fatty deposits in their throat tissue or excess weight in the chest and abdomen that alters breathing.
Age	Muscle tone in the upper airways deteriorates with age.
Sex	Obstructive apnea is more common in men than women.
Event	The airway becomes obstructed during sleep, blocking air flow and resulting in an emergency arousal that causes the person to gasp for air.

Central Sleep Apnea

Central sleep apnea is a rare form that is caused by a problem in the central nervous system. The respiratory center in the brain that is responsible for breathing fails.

Characteristics of Central Sleep Apnea

Characteristic	Description
Snoring	Usually not a symptom
Anatomical Abnormality	No anatomical abnormality
Body Weight	Obstructive apnea in obese individuals can lead to central apnea.
Age	Central apnea may be related to a neurological problem in older adults. Examples include multiple sclerosis (MS), stroke, or amyotrophic lateral sclerosis (ALS or Lou Gehrig's disease).
Sex	Equally as common in men and women.
Event	Breathing stops during sleep when the breathing center in the brain stops working, resulting in an emergency arousal that causes the person to gasp.

Did You Know...
Swollen adenoids can cause snoring.

Mixed Apnea

As the name suggests, mixed apnea is a combination of obstructive and central apnea. Many researchers feel most apnea is a mixed form. The reason for this is because a person with obstructive apnea often has a tendency to breathe rapidly when recovering from an obstructive apnea event, thereby lowering the carbon dioxide level in the blood, which can trigger a central apneic event.

EARLY IDENTIFICATION OF SLEEP APNEA

Excessive sleepiness and snoring in obese patients was identified as sleep apnea as early as 1877. Also known as hypoventilation syndrome, the Pickwickian syndrome is named after a loud-snoring character named Joe in Charles Dickens' book *The Posthumous Papers of the Pickwick Club*. Fat Joe had such excessive trouble with daytime sleepiness, he fell asleep while knocking on a door.

A true Pickwickian is massively obese and has diminished chest wall movement, causing restricted breathing and reduced oxygen intake. This same restricted breathing in a Pickwickian may also lead to carbon dioxide retention, which indirectly results in an increase in red blood cells leading to risks of high blood pressure and possibly heart failure. Pickwickians have severe sleep apnea because of their obesity.

SLEEP APNEA'S SIDE EFFECTS

Statistically, sleep apnea is as prevalent as adult-onset diabetes. According to the National Institute of Health, sleep apnea affects more than twelve million Americans. Untreated sleep apnea can lead to the following:

High Blood Pressure

During apnea events, blood oxygen drops abnormally low, resulting in an increase in blood pressure.

Arrhythmia

Arrhythmia, or abnormal heart rhythm, is very common in people with sleep apnea.

Enlargement of the Heart

People with prolonged episodes of high blood pressure risk enlargement of the heart.

Stroke

High blood pressure and heart enlargement are risk factors associated with stroke.

Lung Dysfunction

Low levels of oxygen in the blood and high concentrations of carbon dioxide can cause abnormalities in lung tissue.

Did You Know…
Breathe Right nasal strips have been approved by the FDA.

SLEEP APNEA AND SUDDEN INFANT DEATH SYNDROME (SIDS)

Although the subject is heavily debated, some experts believe sleep apnea may be a factor in Sudden Infant Death Syndrome or SIDS.

SIDS is a mysterious killer that affects approximately three thousand babies per year in the United States alone. SIDS strikes infants during sleep in their first six months of life, and autopsies show a drastic decrease in oxygen levels.

DOCTORS WHO CAN DIAGNOSE SLEEP APNEA

There are now several categories of specialists who understand sleep and breathing disorders. Examples include the following:

Otolaryngologist

An otolaryngologist is an ear, nose and throat specialist. Doctors who treat the upper air passageways are familiar with sleep apnea because of their training and expertise in nose and throat anatomy.

Pulmonologist or Sleep Specialist

A sleep specialist is usually a pulmonologist with expertise in sleep disorders. Sleep laboratories are usually staffed by pulmonologists.

Neurologist

A neurologist is a doctor who treats neurologic conditions of the brain, spinal cord, and peripheral nerves.

Sometimes these specialties overlap. For example, an otolaryngologist may also be a sleep specialist.

STEPS FOR FINDING A DOCTOR

Your family doctor is likely to be the first person you'll consult about snoring. He/she will probably want to refer you to a specialist, since most medical practitioners are not familiar with sleep disorders.

If you have problems with snoring, daytime sleepiness, fatigue, and insomnia, there's a good chance you have sleep apnea that should be properly evaluated by a specialist who is familiar with sleep disorders. Before drawing any conclusions, a specialist will want to rule out causes such as the following:

- Weight
- Smoking
- Allergies
- Alcohol

He/she may also want you to undergo testing at a sleep laboratory. Most health insurance companies will require an all-night study of sleeping and breathing patterns before they will pay for surgery or other medical treatments for snoring. The test that is used to evaluate snoring and sleep apnea is called a polysomnogram, and the device that's used is called a polysomnograph.

Because you'll need to find a doctor who can help you through simple-to-complex tests to determine the cause of your condition, it's best to find a doctor who has had formal training in the treatment of sleep apnea. Steps for finding a physician and a sleep laboratory include these:

1. Ask your family doctor to refer you to a sleep specialist.

Your family physician may be able to refer you to an otolaryngologist to determine whether there is an anatomic basis for your snoring and decide if testing for sleep apnea is appropriate.

2. Contact the American Academy of Sleep Medicine.

The AASM maintains a list of accredited sleep specialists as well as accredited sleep centers. You may contact them by phone (507-287-6006) or visit their Web site at http://www.aasmnet.org/Listing.htm. Click on the link to your state and browse the list that is organized alphabetically by city (see Chapter 8 for further details).

THE POLYSOMNOGRAM

The polysomnogram has evolved as a standard for measuring sleep. Tests are scheduled in a sleep center, where patients are asked to stay overnight. Sleep laboratories are set up with sleeping rooms that are run by sleep technicians called polysomnographic technologists.

The polysomnograph collects information from electrodes that are taped to a person's head, face, chin, chest, abdomen, and legs. The data that is recorded is then compared to a set of recordings considered to be within normal range. During a polysomnogram session, other monitors are used to record the amount of air traveling in through the nose and mouth as well as the amount of oxygen in the person's blood.

Portable monitoring equipment is a new trend in sleep testing devices. Some home care providers and medical equipment manufacturers have recently expanded their services to include in-home testing. These companies are now supplying the equipment as well as a technician. Careful inquiries should be made in these circumstances to determine if the equipment and services are recommended by the AASM, and covered by your health insurance plan.

MEASURING THE SEVERITY OF APNEA

The Apnea-Hypopnea Index (AHI) has evolved as a measure of severity of apnea. Apnea is a Greek word meaning without breath and hypopnea refers to a breath that is less than normal. While apnea is a complete cessation in breath that may last at least ten seconds, hypopnea is a reduction in airflow. The apnea-hypopnea index is defined as the number of apnea and hypopnea episodes per hour. As a result, the index is calculated by first adding the number of apnea and hypopnea events that occurred while a patient was asleep and then dividing this total by the number of hours of sleep.

Example:
If Harold had a total of 60 apnea episodes and 10 hypopnea episodes during 7 hours of sleep, his AHI index would be:

(60+10)/7
70/7=10

According to the National Institutes of Health's Sleep Heart Health Study (SHHS) reported in the April 12, 2000 issue of the *Journal of the American Medical Association*, sleep apnea is present in patients with an AHI index greater than 5.

Did You Know...
Nasal congestion that can cause snoring is often caused by a cold, hay fever, or a sinus infection. Contact your doctor if your stuffy nose lasts more than two weeks.

Apnea Hypopnea Index (AHI)

Index	Severity
0–5	Normal
6–20	Mild
21–40	Moderate
> 40	Severe

MULTIPLE SLEEP LATENCY TEST (MSLT)

A MSLT test is used to determine the severity of daytime sleepiness. Patients who take this test are usually scheduled for the morning after an all-night polysomnogram. The test usually takes an entire day, and it is designed to measure variations in drowsiness during daytime hours.

Case Study: Stewart

During Stewart's first visit, he reported that he had a long history of severe snoring. His wife, who accompanied him, had urged him to see a doctor because she noticed he appeared to stop breathing at times and also gasped for air during the night. At 57, Stewart complained that he would frequently nod off during the day or while watching television. He also admitted he had generalized fatigue and did not feel rested when he woke up in the morning. Morning headaches were also a problem.

Stewart's Physical Exam

Stewart acknowledged that he had progressively gained weight over the years to reach 225 pounds. Although he denied using alcohol or sedatives regularly, his wife volunteered that his sleep pattern was worse after he socialized and had cocktails. Stewart also had a history of hypertension and was being treated for his high blood pressure.

A physical exam revealed Stewart to be moderately obese, and a nasal exam revealed a mildly deviated septum even though Stewart denied symptoms of chronic nasal obstruction. A throat exam revealed enlarged tonsils, a large uvula, and crowding of the soft tissues at the back of his throat. An exam of the lower part of his throat was normal.

Sleep Apnea

At the conclusion of Stewart's physical exam, a provisional diagnosis of obstructive sleep apnea was made based on physical findings and his wife's description of his symptoms during sleep. To confirm the diagnosis, Stewart was referred to a local sleep diagnostic center for an overnight sleep study. Two weeks later, at Stewart's follow-up visit to review the sleep study results, his respiratory disturbance index was 58—a score that is consistent with severe obstructive sleep apnea. Various treatment options were reviewed and a nasal Continuous Positive Airway Pressure (CPAP) device was recommended.

CPAP—The Gold Standard

A CPAP device is a small portable generator that pushes air though the nose and into the upper airways to hold the tissues apart. The generator sends air through a hose and into a p astic mask that covers the nose. The CPAP device is the gold standard for treatment of obstructive sleep apnea because of its effectiveness. An appointment was made for Stewart to return to the sleep laboratory to be fitted for a CPAP mask and receive instruction on how to use the equipment.

At a follow-up consultation six weeks later, Stewa t described his initial difficulties adjusting to the CPAP device. They eventually subsided, and his wife reported that his sleep patterns were much more normal with almost no snoring. Stewart repo ted feeling well rested with increased energy during the day. With an increase in energy, he made a commitment to a diet and regular exercise. His goal is to lose weight so that he can discontinue use of the CPAP

7

Treatment for Snoring and Sleep Apnea

Although snoring and obstructive sleep apnea are related conditions, the approach to treatment varies significantly. Snoring is not generally considered to be a medical problem by the public, and treatment is optional (although sleeping partners of snorers may believe otherwise!).

Obstructive sleep apnea is considered a medical condition with long-term adverse effects on the cardiovascular system because of the repeated lowering of blood oxygen levels throughout the night, increasing the work of the heart. As a result, treatment for obstructive sleep apnea, especially when severe, should not be considered optional. Treatment for severe obstructive sleep apnea should be considered necessary to optimum health, much like treatment for high blood pressure.

TREATMENT FOR SNORING: LIFESTYLE MODIFICATION

Lifestyle modification is considered to be the best first step in the treatment of snoring and includes the following:

Weight Loss

Excess weight is the most common contributing factor. Individuals who are even mildly overweight can significantly reduce their snoring with a very modest weight loss of five to ten pounds.

Smoking

Because smoking leads to irritation and dryness of mucous membranes, the elimination of cigars or cigarettes is a lifestyle change that can have a dramatic impact on snoring

Alcohol, Sedatives, and Sedating Antihistamines

Alcohol, sedatives, and sedating antihistamines lower muscle tone in the upper airways, causing an increased airway resistance and snoring. Many people who reduce these substances report improvements in their snoring.

Sleep Position

For some people, an increased amount of obstruction occurs when they sleep on their backs. Described as positional snoring, this type of snoring explains a snorer's common complaint of being "frequently assaulted" through the night and implored to roll over. A simple remedy is to sew a ball into the pocket of a T-shirt that is then worn backward during sleep, keeping the snorer off of his/her back. Some positional snorers also improve when the head of the bed is elevated.

TREATMENT FOR SNORING: CLEARING NASAL PASSAGEWAYS

Treating nasal obstruction and congestion, which often solves a snoring problem that is related to upper airway obstruction, includes the following:

Identification and Avoidance of Allergens

Nasal allergies, which are either seasonal or perennial, increase nasal congestion. Numerous treatments are available to provide identification and avoidance of allergens. For example, dust allergies are common, and exposure can be reduced with the use of nonallergenic bedding, removal of carpeting or upholstery, and the use of an air cleaner with a High Efficiency Particulate Air (HEPA) filter.

Treatment for Nasal Allergies

Several medications are available for the treatment of nasal allergies, including the following:

- **Nasal Crom** is an over-the-counter nasal spray that reduces the release of histamine in the nose.
- **Prescription Nasal Steroid Sprays** decrease allergic and nonallergic inflammation in the nose and can be safely used for a long period of time.
- **Nonsedating Antihistamines** can reduce allergic nasal congestion when used alone or with a nasal spray.
- **Allergy Injections** are for patients with long-standing identifiable allergies (that may be identified through skin or blood tests). Allergy injections gradually reduce symptoms and the need for medication.

Treatment for Chronic Sinusitis

Chronic sinusitis is a common condition associated with nasal obstruction that will lead to increased snoring. Symptoms include chronic nasal congestion, facial pain, headaches, nasal discharge, and postnasal drip. Treatment options include the following:

- **Antibiotic Therapy.** Combined with decongestants and/or nasal steroid spray, antibiotic therapy is sometimes an effective way to eliminate chronic sinusitis.
- **Endoscopic Sinus Surgery.** For those who do not respond to antibiotic therapy, a CAT scan of the sinuses is used to confirm chronic sinusitis. Endoscopic sinus surgery may be used to drain the sinuses.

Treatment for Nasal Polyps

Nasal polyps are a possible cause of chronic nasal obstruction. Individuals with nasal polyps experience progressive nasal blockage and a diminished sense of smell. Often, polyps occur in people who have environmental allergies and/or asthma. Treatment options include the following:

- **Oral Steroids.** Oral steroids such as prednisone will temporarily shrink polyps and improve symptoms.
- **Polyp Removal.** Long-term relief from polyps requires surgery to remove the polyps and reopen the nasal airways. Patients with nasal polyps should undergo an allergy evaluation, since allergies need to be treated to prevent the regrowth of polyps.

Treatment for Deviated Nasal Septum

The most common cause of nasal obstruction is a deviation of the nasal septum. It may be present at birth or arise as the result of nasal trauma. Symptoms include unilateral (one side), bilateral (both sides), or alternating obstruction; postnasal drip; recurrent nose bleeds; and snoring. Breathing usually improves when the cheeks are pulled back speading the nose open. Use of over-the-counter decongestant nasal sprays will improve breathing but should be avoided because prolonged use leads to increased mucosal inflammation and obstruction. More appropriate treatment options include the following:

- **Dilator Nasal Strips (Breathe Right).** These dilator nasal strips may alleviate symptoms of obstruction that are caused by a deviated nasal septum. When the strips are worn at bedtime, patients with a mild or moderate deviated septum may find their snoring is decreased. There are no contraindications to the use of dilator nasal strips. If they are effective, they can be used indefinitely for the treatment of snoring.

- **Surgical Correction of a Deviated Nasal Septum.** Permanent relief of nasal obstruction and snoring caused by a deviated nasal septum requires surgical correction. Called a septoplasty, or submucous resection, this procedure is performed in an outpatient setting under local or general anesthesia. All incisions are made inside the nose. Although there is temporary nasal congestion following surgery, patients generally do not experience pain. There is no external swelling or black-and-blue bruising unless cosmetic nasal surgery was also performed. Commonly, to augment an improvement in the nasal airway, a reduction of the inferior nasal turbinates is also performed in conjunction with nasal septal surgery. The most common complication in nasal septal and turbinate surgery is bleeding, which requires the placement of additional nasal packing.

- **Oral Appliances.** These are designed to move the lower jaw out and the tongue forward to enlarge the airway. They may be purchased over the counter or custom fitted by a dentist. Potential problems with oral appliances include jaw pain and drooling.

TREATMENT FOR SNORING: SOLUTIONS IN THE THROAT

Once lifestyle modifications have been considered and tried, and nasal airway issues have been satisfactorily addressed, treatment of snoring is targeted to the soft tissue in the back of the throat. The loud noise associated with snoring comes from vibration of the soft palate and uvula. Successful reduction of snoring requires reducing the vibration of these structures, including the following:

Removal of Enlarged Tonsils, or Tonsillectomy

If large tonsils are present, they should be removed or reduced in size. Conventional tonsillectomy is effective, but this procedure is associated with seven to ten days of postoperative throat pain and the risk of hemorrhage. Newer techniques are available to reduce the size of the tonsils without removing them, decreasing postoperative pain and bleeding risk.

Trimming the Uvula and Soft Palate, or Laser-Assisted Uvulopalatopharyngoplasty (LAUP)

A popular treatment for snoring is laser-assisted uvulopalatopharyngoplasty(LAUP). Usually performed in a doctor's office with local anesthesia, LAUP involves the use of a laser to trim the uvula and create "trenches" in the soft palate to enlarge the pharyngeal airway. In many cases, LAUP is performed as a staged procedure, requiring two or three sessions separated by six-week intervals. Although often successful, LAUP is associated with significant postprocedure pain, and a possible residual sensation of dryness in the throat.

Reducing the Vibration of Soft Tissue, or Radio-frequency Palatoplasty

A more recent and less invasive treatment for snoring is radio-frequency palatoplasty. Performed in the doctor's office with local anesthesia, a radio-frequency probe is inserted into the soft palate, where it delivers heat that causes inflammation and scarring, reducing the vibration of the soft tissue. Discomfort following the procedure is mild, and it is treated with acetaminophen and throat lozenges. If snoring is not significantly reduced, a second radio-frequency procedure may be successful. In addition to convenience and comfort, another advantage of the radio-frequency procedure is that because no tissue is removed, there is no permanent change in throat sensation.

Stiffening the Soft Palate, or Injection Snoreplasty

The newest procedure for the treatment of snoring is injection snoreplasty. Performed in the doctor's office, a small amount of medication is injected beneath the surface of the soft palate. This medication had originally been developed for the treatment of varicose veins. Injection of the material into the vein caused scarring and shrinkage of the varicosity. Doctors found that the same medication could be safely injected into the soft palate. A local inflammatory reaction causes scarring that increases the stiffness of the palate, resulting in less snoring. Once again, discomfort following the procedure is mild, and there are no long-term side effects. A second injection snoreplasty may be performed if the result following the first procedure is not acceptable.

TREATMENT FOR SLEEP APNEA: LIFESTYLE MODIFICATION

Treatment of obstructive sleep apnea should initially focus on lifestyle modification. Excessive weight is the most common risk factor, and a weight loss program, combining diet and exercise, should be pursued.

The use of alcohol and/or sedatives, particularly in the late evening, should be discontinued, since they lower muscle tone and increase obstruction. Smokers should be strongly advised to stop smoking. In addition to the well-documented adverse effects of smoking, chronic irritation and drying of the air passageways lead to increased obstruction.

TREATMENT FOR SLEEP APNEA: BREATHING DEVICES

Breathing devices worn at night are designed to keep tissues from collapsing. Examples include the following:

Continuous Positive Airway Pressure (CPAP)

The gold standard for the treatment of obstructive sleep apnea is continuous positive airway pressure, or CPAP. A CPAP unit delivers a continuous flow of air through the upper respiratory tract and acts as a stent, keeping the tissues from collapsing. The CPAP unit consists of a small air pressure generator connected by tubing to a snug-fitting nasal mask that is worn while sleeping.

Although extremely effective, compliance with the use of CPAP units is also a significant issue. Many people are uncomfortable sleeping with the nasal mask, and they describe a claustrophobic feeling. Humidifying equipment attached to CPAP units reduces the sensation of throat dryness. Also, individuals with significant nasal congestion may require treatment of their underlying nasal condition to comfortably tolerate the nasal mask.

For those with moderate to severe obstructive sleep apnea who are unwilling or unable to tolerate CPAP, surgical intervention is the remaining option. A variety of procedures are available, but most offer limited success rates, generally in the range of 50 percent. The choice of procedure is based on individual anatomic considerations, such as size of the tonsils or tongue base.

Bilevel Positive Airway Pressure (BiPAP)

A similar device, bilevel positive airway pressure, or BiPAP, delivers pressurized air flow only during the inspiration. CPAP and BiPAP units are customized to the individual's needs by respiratory therapists. Proper fit of the nasal mask is necessary, and appropriate air pressure settings should be established for each individual. The units are portable and may be used when traveling.

TREATMENT FOR SLEEP APNEA: SURGERY

After other treatments have been considered and tried, the treatment of obstructive sleep apnea may include the following surgical procedures:

Uvulopalatopharyngoplasty, or UPPP

The most common surgical procedure for obstructive sleep apnea is the uvulopalatopharyngoplasty or UPPP. Performed under general anesthesia, UPPP is performed by removing the uvula and a small portion of the soft palate. If enlarged tonsils are present, they will be removed at the same time. The procedure causes considerable throat pain, especially when combined with tonsillectomy, which may last up to two weeks. Postoperative bleeding from the throat is a potential complication. After recovering from a UPPP, some patients describe a sensation of dryness or phlegm in the back of throat, which is related to the absence of the uvula. A rare complication occurs when too much of the soft palate is removed, leading to regurgitation of liquids through the nose.

Often, individuals with obstructive sleep apnea have concurrent nasal obstruction, which contributes to their condition. Many physicians will surgically correct a deviated nasal septum and/or reduce the size of the turbinates at the same time as performing a UPPP.

The best candidates for UPPP are patients whose tonsils can be visualized when they open their mouths fully. This reduces the possibility that a large tongue is the primary source of obstruction. Although short-term results following UPPP have been encouraging, in some individuals scarring produces narrowing of the airway, leading to recurrent obstruction.

Genioglossal Advancement and Hyoid Suspension

For patients who do not improve following UPPP, or are not candidates for UPPP, maxillofacial surgical techniques have been developed to reduce airway obstruction at the base of the tongue, below the level of the palate and tonsils. Candidates for these procedures have severe obstructive sleep apnea, and usually have a short, thick neck.

Genioglossal advancement pulls the base of the tongue forward by repositioning a muscle attached to the tongue. Hyoid suspension lifts the tongue and pulls it forward, opening the airway at the base of the tongue. The most radical surgical option for repositioning the tongue is maxillomandibular advancement, when the bones of the upper and lower jaw are cut and moved forward with the use of surgical plates and screws.

Tracheotomy

The ultimate surgical treatment for severe obstructive sleep apnea that has the highest success rate is tracheotomy. A surgical opening is created in the windpipe, through which a tracheotomy tube is placed. Because air flows directly into the trachea, bypassing the pharyngeal tissues and tongue, obstruction is eliminated. Tracheotomy, requiring significant lifestyle adaptation, is generally reserved for morbidly obese patients who are at risk for the complications associated with severe obstructive sleep apnea.

TREATMENT FOR SLEEP APNEA IN CHILDREN

Fortunately, the evaluation and treatment of obstructive sleep apnea in children is much simpler than in adults. In children, the cause of obstruction is enlarged tonsils, adenoids, or both. Removal of the tonsils and/or adenoids is a safe outpatient procedure. Children will experience a sore throat for one week following surgery, and there is a very small risk of postoperative bleeding. The success rate is almost 100 percent, and in most cases, the child will stop snoring immediately following surgery.

Case Study: Robert

At 42, Robert's loud snoring caused his wife to insist that he sleep in their guest room, and it was her prompting that made him seek treatment. During his initial visit, Robert denied that he had daytime fatigue, sleepiness, or frequent headaches. When asked about a recent weight gain or the regular use of alcohol, Robert claimed neither pertained to him. Although Robert's past medical history was negative, he reported that he had had his tonsils and adenoids removed as a child. He also admitted to a long history of nonseasonal nasal obstruction.

Robert's Deviated Nasal Septum

Physically, Robert is a tall, thin man. An examination of his nose revealed a severely deviated septum with no polyps or sign of infection. In addition, his throat showed that his tonsils had been removed, and there was no evidence of crowding of soft tissue in the back of his throat. His remaining airway passages were also normal. When Robert's history and physical findings were reviewed, it was concluded that significant sleep apnea was not likely. It was suggested that his snoring was due to a deviated nasal septum and that treatment be aimed at his nasal obstruction. As a conservative first step, a nasal steroid spray was prescribed, and Robert was asked to purchase nasal breathing strips to use while sleeping.

The Need for Surgery

Three weeks later, Robert returned for a consultation and reported that his wife had not noticed any change in his snoring and that his nasal obstruction had only minimally improved. Because Robert did not respond to the nasal spray and breathing strips, a turbinectomy and surgery to repair his deviated nasal septum were recommended.

The nasal septum is a structure that ordinarily divides the nasal cavity in half. In Robert's case, a deviated or crooked septum blocked his air passageways. A deviated septum may be present from birth or it may be caused by damage to the nose from a fight or a fall. Repairing a deviated septum involves moving or repositioning cartilage and bone.

The nasal turbinates are bulky structures that occupy a large space within the nasal cavity. Covered by mucous membranes that protrude into the nasal airway, they can become chronically enlarged, producing symptoms of nasal obstruction or a stuffy nose. Turbinectomy refers to a procedure in which a portion of the turbinates is removed to enlarge the airway.

Both surgeries were easily accomplished on an outpatient basis. However, six weeks following the surgery, Robert reported that although his nasal obstruction had significantly improved, his wife still heard snoring and continued her request that he sleep in a different room. A sleep study to exclude the possibility of significant sleep apnea was selected as the next course of action, and portable monitoring equipment was arranged at Robert's home.

Sleep Study Results
Robert's sleep study results revealed a respiratory disturbance index of 5, which confirmed that he did not have sleep apnea. During his visit to review the sleep study results, various other treatment options were discussed, including uvulopalatopharyngoplasty, laser-assisted uvulopalatoplasty, radio-frequency palatoplasty, and snoreplasty. After discussing the various treatment options with his wife, Robert decided to schedule a snoreplasty.

Robert's Injection Snoreplasty
Robert's injection snoreplasty was performed in the office, and he was able to work the following day. During a follow-up visit two weeks later, he described a mild sore throat immediately following the snoreplasty that had lasted a few days. A throat exam revealed a shallow healing ulcer of the soft palate. One month after the snoreplasty, Robert reported that while his snoring had not completely disappeared, its volume was lower and the improvement made it possible for his wife to sleep in the same bed. A throat exam revealed a small midline dimple in the soft palate.

8

Resources

Although very little was known about snoring and sleep apnea for many years, there are now world conferences and scientific studies that provide much-needed information on effective treatments.

This chapter provides information about sleep support groups, sleep organizations in the United States and Europe, universities with programs in sleep medicine, board-certified sleep specialists, and accredited sleep centers. Sleep centers, sleep organizations, and sleep support groups provide information and outreach for people with apnea and those who are yet to be diagnosed.

SUPPORT GROUPS

The following list includes nonprofit organizations dedicated to sleep disorders:

THE A.W.A.K.E. NETWORK

Alert, Well, And Keeping Energetic
Mutual-Help Support Groups
for Persons Affected by Sleep Apnea
202-293-3650
awake@sleepapnea.org.

Wake Up America

701 Welch Road, Suite 2226
Palo Alto, California 94304
650-725-6484
http://www.stanford.edu/~dement/wua.html

SLEEP ORGANIZATIONS IN THE UNITED STATES

The following list includes nonprofit organizations dedicated to sleep disorders:

American Sleep Apnea Association

1424 K Street NW, Suite 302
Washington, DC 20005
202-293-3650
Fax: 202-293-3656
http://www.sleepapnea.org
asaa@sleepapnea.org

The National Sleep Foundation

1522 K Street, NW, Suite 500
Washington, DC 20005
202-347-3471
Fax 202-347-3472
http://www.sleepfoundation.org
nsf@sleepfoundation.org

Sleep Disorders Dental Society (SDDS)

10592 Perry Highway #220
Building 1, Suite 1204
Wexford, PA 15090-0224
724-935-0836
http://www.thesdds.org

Sleep Research Society

708-492-1093
http://www.sleepresearchsociety.org

INTERNATIONAL SLEEP ORGANIZATIONS

The following list includes international nonprofit organizations dedicated to sleep disorders:

British Sleep Society

P.O. Box 247
Huntingdon PE28 3UZ
UK
Martin.KING@papworth-tr.anglox.nhs.uk

The Sleep Apnoea Trust (United Kingdom)

7 Bailey Close
High Wycombe
HP13 6QA
United Kingdom
Tel :+44 (0)1494 527772
http://www.sleepmatters.org/

Sleep/Wake Disorders Canada

5385 Yonge Street
P. O. Box 45034
North York, ON M2N 5R7
Tel: 416-483-9654
Fax: 416-483-7081
http://swdca.org
swdc@globalserve.net

Canadian Sleep Society

3080 Yonge Street., Ste 5055/3080, rue Yonge, Bureau 5055,
Toronto, ON, Canada, M4N 3N1
tel. 416-483-6260, fax 416-483-7081
http://www.css.to/

Sleep Apnea Society of Alberta

283-1559 in the Calgary region
1-800-81-SLEEP (75337) outside Calgary.
http://www.sleep-apnea.ab.ca/
sasa@sleep-apnea.ab.ca.

Finnish Sleep Research Society

Secretary Outi Saarenpää-Heikkilä
TAYS, Children's clinic
PO Box 2000, 33521
Tampere, Finland
Phone:+358 3 247 7526
http://www.sus.fi/index-en.html
email: klousa@uta.fi

Irish Sleep Apnoea Trust

PO BOX 8440
Dublin 24
Ireland
Tel. International+353 (86) 605 3891
Tel National (086) 605 3891
http://www.isat.ie

European Sleep Research Society

Institute of Biomedicine, University of Helsinki
Biomedicum, P.O.B. 63
FIN-00014 Helsinki, Finland
phone:+358-9-191 25317
fax+358-9-191 25302
http://www.esrs.org/
porkka@cc.helsinki.fi

German Sleep Society (DGSM)

PD Dr. Thomas Penzel
Klinikum der Philipps-Universität Marburg
Baldingerstraße D-35033 Marburg
penzel@mailer.uni-marburg.de

UNIVERSITIES AND HOSPITALS WITH PROGRAMS IN SLEEP MEDICINE

The following list includes universities that have AASM-accredited fellowship programs in sleep disorders medicine:

Stanford, CA

Stanford University
Stanford Sleep Disorders Clinic
401 Quarry Road
Suite 3301
Stanford, CA 94305-5547
Phone: 650-723-6601/415-725-5911
Fax: 650-725-8910
Program Director: Christian
Guilleminault, MD

Denver, CO

National Jewish Medical and Research
Center/University of Colorado Health
Sciences Center
Sleep Health Centers at National Jewish
1400 Jackson Street
Denver, CO 80206
Phone: 303-398-1523
Fax: 303-270-2109
Program Director: Robert D. Ballard,
MD

Miami Beach, FL

Mount Sinai Sleep Disorders Center
4300 Alton Road
Miami Beach, FL 33140
Phone: 305-674-2613
Fax: 305-674-2647
Program Director: Alejandro D.
Chediak, MD

Chicago, IL

The University of Chicago
Sleep Disorders Center
5841 S. Maryland Avenue, MC3077
Chicago, IL 60637
Phone: 773-702-6531

Fax: 773-702-7998
Program Director: Jean-Paul Spire, MD

Chicago, IL

Children's Memorial Hospital
Sleep Medicine Center
2300 Children's Plaza
Box 43
Chicago, IL 60614
Phone: 773-880-8230
Fax: 773-880-4057
Program Director: Stephen H. Sheldon,
DO

Chicago, IL

Rush-Presbyterian-St. Luke's Medical
Center-PhD Route
Sleep Disorders Center
1653 West Congress Parkway
Chicago, IL 60612-3833
Phone: 312-942-5440
Fax: 312-942-8961
Program Director: Edward J. Stepanski,
PhD

Chicago, IL

Rush-Presbyterian-St. Luke's Medical
Center
Sleep Disorders Center
1653 West Congress Parkway
Chicago, IL 60612-3833
Phone: 312-942-5440
Fax: 312-942-8961
Program Director: Damien R. Stevens,
MD and James J. Herdegen, MD

Chicago, IL

Northwestern University Medical
School

Department of Neurology
710 North Lakeshore Drive
Suite 1126
Chicago, IL 60611
Phone: 312-908-8549
Fax: 312-908-5073
Program Director: Phyllis C. Zee, MD,
PhD

Indianapolis, IN

Sleep Medicine and Circadian Biology
Program/Indiana University School of
Medicine
Department of Medicine
550 N. University Boulevard
University Hospital/UH5450
Indianapolis, IN 46202
Phone: 317-274-2136
Fax: 317-274-4224
Program Director: Brian H. Foresman,
DO, FCCP

Lexington, KY

University of Kentucky
MN-614, UKMC
800 Rose Street
Lexington, KY 40536-0084
Phone: 859-323-5419
Fax: 859-323-1020
Program Director: Barbara Phillips, MD

Boston, MA

Brigham & Women's Hospital
221 Longwood Avenue
RFB 486
Boston, MA 02115
Phone: 617-732-5778
Fax: 617-975-0809
Program Director: David White, MD

Brighton, MA

St. Elizabeths Medical Center
736 Cambridge Street
Brighton, MA 02135
Phone: 617-789-2545
Program Director. Edwin M. Trayner,
Jr., MD

Burlington, MA

Lahey Clinic
41 Mall Road
Burlington, MA 01805
Phone: 781-744-8480
Fax: 781-744-3443
Program Director: David Neumeyer,
MD

Worcester, MA

Worcester Medical Center Campus at
St. Vincent Hospital
Department of Neurology
20 Worcester Center Boulevard
Worcester, MA 01608
Phone: 508-363-6066
Fax: 508-363-6373
Program Director: Jayant Phadke, MD

Ann Arbor, MI

Michael S. Aldrich Sleep Disorders
Laboratory
UH 8D8702-0117
University of Michigan Medical Center
1500 East Medical Center Drive
Ann Arbor, MI 48109-0117
Phone: 734-647-5064
Fax: 734-647-9065
Program Director: Beth Malow, MD

Detroit, MI

VA Medical Center
Sleep/Wake Disorders Unit (127B)
4646 John R
Detroit, MI 48201
Phone: 313-966-0695
Fax: 313-745-2481
Program Director: Sheldon Kapen, MD
and M. Safwan Badr, MD

Detroit, MI

Henry Ford Hospital
HFH Sleep Disorders & Research
Center
2799 W. Grand Boulevard
CFP-3
Detroit, MI 48202-2691
Phone: 313-916-4417
Fax: 313-916-5150
Program Director: David Hudgel, MD

Rochester, MN

Mayo Sleep Disorders Center
Mayo Clinic
200 First St SW
Rochester, MN 55905
Phone: 507-266-8900
Fax: 507-255-6506
Program Director: Lois E. Krahn, MD

Jackson, MS

University of Mississippi Medical
Center
Sleep Disorders Center
2500 North State Street
Jackson, MS 39216-4505
Phone: 601-984-4820
Fax: 601-984-4828
Program Director: Allen Richert, MD

Durham, NC

Duke University Medical Center
DUMC
Box 3678
202 Bell Building
Durham, NC 27710
Phone: 919-684-8485
Fax: 919-684-8955
Program Director: Aatif Husain, MD

Omaha, NE

University of Nebraska Medical Center
(UNMC)
Box 985300 Nebraska Medical Center
Omaha, NE 68198-5300
Phone: 402-559-4087
Fax: 402-559-8210
Program Director: Teri J. Bowman, MD

Edison, NJ

Seton Hall University School of
Graduate Medical Education
Center for Sleep Disorders Treatment
Research and Education
65 James Street
Edison, NJ 08818
Phone: 732-321-7000 x68177
Program Director: Arthur S. Walters,
MD

Newark, NJ

Newark Beth Israel Sleep Disorders
Center
201 Lyons Avenue
Newark, NJ 07112
Phone: 973-926-7163
Fax: 973-282-0821
Program Director: Jeffrey Nahmias, MD

Albuquerque, NM

New Mexico Center for Sleep Medicine
4700 Jefferson NE
Suite 800
Albuquerque, NM 87109
Phone: 505-872-6000
Fax: 505-872-6003
Program Director: John Doggett, MD

Buffalo, NY

SUNY Buffalo School of Medicine
Department of Medicine
100 High Street
Buffalo, NY 14203
Phone: 716-859-2271
Fax: 716-859-1491
Program Director: Eric Ten Brock, MD

Manhasset, NY

North Shore University Hospital
Division of Pulmonary and Critical
Care Medicine
300 Community Drive
Manhasset, NY 11030
Phone: 516-465-8270
Fax: 516-562-4908
Program Director: Steven Feinsilver,
MD

New Hyde Park, NY

Long Island Jewish Medical Center
Division of Pulmonary and Critical
Care Medicine
270-05 76th Avenue
New Hyde Park, NY 11040
Phone: 516-470-6400
Fax: 516-488-7162
Program Director: Harly Greenberg,
MD

Stony Brook, NY

Center for the Study of Sleep and
Waking
SUNY Stony Brook
University Hospital MR 120-A
Stony Brook, NY 11794-7139
Phone: 631-444-2916
Fax: 631-444-7851
Program Director. Marta Maczaj, MD

Cleveland, OH

Cleveland Clinic Foundation
Sleep Disorders Center
9500 Euclid Avenue, S-51
Cleveland, OH 44195
Phone: 216-445-2990
Fax: 216-445-6205
Program Director: Nancy Foldvary, DO

Cleveland, OH

Case Western Reserve University
111j(w) VAMC
10701 East Boulevard
Cleveland, OH 44106
Phone: 216-231-3399
Fax: 216-231-3475/3420
Program Director: Kingman P. Strohl,
MD, Carol Rosen, MD,
and Dennis Auckley, MD

Philadelphia, PA

University of Pennsylvania
Sleep Medicine Fellowship Program
991 Maloney
3600 Spruce Street
Philadelphia, PA 19104
Phone: 215-662-3305
Fax: 215-662-7749
Program Director: Samuel T. Kuna, MD

Pittsburgh, PA

University of Pittsburgh School of
Medicine
Psychiatry and Medicine, Division of
Pulmonary
3811 O'Hara Street
Room E1127
Pittsburgh, PA 15213
Phone: 412-624-2246
Fax: 412-624-2841
Program Director: Daniel Buysse, MD
and Patrick J. Strollo, Jr, MD

Dallas, TX

University of Texas Southwestern
Medical Center
5323 Harry Hines Boulevard
Dallas, TX 75390-9182
Phone: 214-456-7267
Program Dir.: John H. Herman, PhD
Email:

Temple, TX

Scott & White Memorial Hospital and
Clinic
2401 South 31st Street
Temple, TX 76508
Phone: 254-724-2554
Fax: 254-724-2497
Program Director: James A. Barker, MD

Salt Lake City, UT

Intermountain Sleep Disorders Center
at LDS Hospital
8th Avenue & C Street
Salt Lake City, UT 84143
Phone: 801-408-3617
Fax: 801-408-5110
Program Director: Tom V. Cloward,
MD, Robert J. Farney, MD, and James
M. Walker, PhD

SLEEP SPECIALISTS

The American Academy of Sleep Medicine (AASM) sets standards for professionalism in the field of sleep medicine. AASM members are accredited sleep centers and sleep specialists. At present, there are more than one thousand board-certified sleep specialists in the United States.

The AASM has two branches of membership, Center Members and Individual Members. The center membership branch encompasses **AASM-accredited centers and laboratories** that have elected to make a membership commitment to the academy in order to further advance the field. The individual member branch includes clinicians involved in the diagnosis and treatment of patients with disorders of sleep.

The American Academy of Sleep Medicine
One Westbrook Corporate Center, Suite 920
Westchester, IL 60154
Phone: 708-492-0930
Fax: 708-492-0943
http://www.aasmnet.org/
Email: **cpulvino@aasmnet.org**

SLEEP CENTERS

An asterisk (*) denotes an accredited sleep disorders laboratory for
sleep-related breathing disorders; all other programs are accredited full-
service sleep disorders centers.

Alabama

Albertville

Sleep Disorders Center
Marshall Medical Center
11491 Highway 431
Suite E
Albertville, AL 35950
Phone: 256-891-7806
Fax: 256-891-1147
E-mail: **lori.johnson@mmcs.org**

Anniston

Sleep Disorders Laboratory*
Northeast Alabama Regional Medical
Center
400 East 10th Street
PO Box 2208
Anniston, AL 36202
Phone: 256-235-5077
Fax: 256-231-8813

Athens

Athens-Limestone Hospital
700 West Market Street
PO Box 999
Athens, AL 35611
Phone: 256-233-9240
Fax: 256-233-9575
E-mail:
cherwal@respiratory.alhosp.org

Birmingham

Sleep/Wake Disorders Center
Princeton Baptist Medical Center
817 Princeton Avenue SW
POB II, Suite 61
Birmingham, AL 35211-1399
Phone: 205-783-7378
Fax: 205-783-7386
Web Site: **www.BHSALA.COM**

Birmingham

CMMC Sleep Disorders Center
Carraway Methodist Medical Center
1600 Carraway Boulevard
Birmingham, AL 35234
Phone: 205-502-6164
Fax: 205-502-5210
E-mail: **JERICBARG@AOL.COM**

Birmingham

Brookwood Sleep Disorders Center
Brookwood Medical Center
2010 Brookwood Medical Center Drive
Birmingham, AL 35209
Phone: 205-877-2403
Fax: 205-877-1663

Birmingham

Sleep-Wake Disorders Center
University of Alabama at Birmingham
1713 6th Avenue South
CPM Building, Room 270
Birmingham, AL 35233-0018
Phone: 205-934-7110
Fax: 205-934-6870
E-mail: **lshigley@uabmc.edu**

Birmingham

Sleep Disorders Center of Alabama, Inc.
790 Montclair Road
Suite 200
Birmingham, AL 35213
Phone: 205-599-1020
Fax: 205-599-1029
Web Site: **www.sleepsciences.com**

Birmingham

Sleep Disorders Center
at HealthSouth Medical Center
1201 11th Avenue South
Birmingham, AL 35205
Phone: 205-599-1020
Fax: 205-599-1029
E-mail: **jilluck@sleepsciences.com**

Cullman

Sleep Disorders Center/
Neurodiagnostic Lab
Cullman Regional Medical Center
1912 Alabama Highway 157
Cullman, AL 35056-1108
Phone: 256-737-2140
Fax: 256-737-2261
Web Site: **www.crmc-bhs.com/
services/sleep/sleep.htm**

Decatur

Decatur General Sleep Disorders
Center
1201 Seventh Street SE
PO Box 2239
Decatur, AL 35609-3337
Phone: 256-340-2558
Fax: 256-340-2566

Dothan

Sleep-Wake Disorders Center
Flowers Hospital
4370 West Main Street
PO Box 6907
Dothan, AL 36305
Phone: 334-793-5000 x1685
Fax: 334-615-7213
E-mail: **RCKinALA@aol.com**

Fairfield

Sleep Disorders Lab
Healthsourth Metro West Hospital
701 Richard M. Scrushy Parkway
Fairfield, AL 35064
Phone: 205-783-5576
Fax: 205-783-5578
E-mail:
aneshia.williams@healthsouth.com

Fairhope

Thomas Hospital Sleep Services*
Thomas Hospital
188 Hospital Drive
Suite 201
Fairhope, AL 36532
Phone: 334-990-1940
Fax: 334-990-1941
E-mail:
dmccoy@ThomasHospital.com

Gadsden

Sleep Diagnostics of Northeast Alabama
for Breathing Related Disorders
at Gadsden Regional Medical Center
1007 Goodyear Avenue
Gadsden, AL 35903
Phone: 256-494-4551
Fax: 256-494-4602

Huntsville

The Crestwood Center for Sleep
Disorders
250 Chateau Drive
Suite 235
Huntsville, AL 35801
Phone: 256-880-4710
Fax: 256-880-4708

Huntsville

The Sleep Center at Huntsville Hospital
911 Big Cove
Huntsville, AL 35801
Phone: 256-517-8553
Fax: 256-517-8338
E-mail: **paull@md.hhsys.org**

Jacksonville

Jacksonville Sleep Lab &
Neurodiagnostics*
1701 Pelham Road South
PO Box 999
Jacksonville, AL 36265
Phone: 256-782-4685
Fax: 256-782-4694
E-mail: **solson@jaxhosp.com**

Jasper

Walker Baptist Sleep Disorders Center
Walker Baptist Medical Center
3400 Hwy 78E
Jasper, AL 35501
Phone: 205-387-4461
Fax: 205-387-4681

Mobile

USA Knollwood Sleep Disorders
Center
University of South Alabama
Knollwood Park Hospital
5644 Girby Road
Mobile, AL 36693-3398
Phone: 251-660-5757
Fax: 251-660-5254
E-mail: **wbrought@usouthal.edu**

Mobile

Sleep Apnea Center*
Providence Hospital
6801 Airport Boulevard
Mobile, AL 36608
Phone: 251-639-2876
Fax: 251-639-2999
E-mail:
nwhitele@providencehospital.org

Mobile

Sleep Disorders Center
Mobile Infirmary Medical Center
PO Box 2144
Mobile, AL 36652
Phone: 251-435-5559 or 800-422-2027
Fax: 251-435-5222
Web Site: **www.mimc.com/sleep.html**

Mobile

Southeast Regional Center for Sleep/
Wake Disorders
Springhill Memorial Hospital
3719 Dauphin Street
Mobile, AL 36608
Phone: 251-460-5319
Fax: 251-460-5464

Montgomery

Sleep Disorders Center
Baptist Medical Center South
2105 East South Boulevard
Montgomery, AL 36116-2498
Phone: 334-286-3252
Fax: 334-286-3108
E-mail: **TCTaylor@Baptistfirst.org**

Montgomery

Jackson Sleep Disorders Center
Jackson—MedSouth
1722 Pine Street
Suite 300
Montgomery, AL 36106
Phone: 888-454-9067
Fax: 334-264-0295
E-mail: **CaryCLAE@aol.com**
Web Site: **medsouthinc.net**

Opelika

East Alabama Sleep Disorders Center
East Alabama Medical Center
2000 Pepperell Parkway
Opelika, AL 36801-5452
Phone: 334-705-2404
Fax: 334-705-2403
E-mail: **gina_white@eamc.org**
Web Site: **www.eamc.org**

Scottsboro

The Sleep Center at Jackson County
Hospital
380 Woods Cove Road
Scottsboro, AL 35768
Phone: 256-218-3639
Fax: 256-218-3607
E-mail: **sleeper45@msn.com**

Sheffield

North Alabama Sleep Disorders Center
Helen Keller Hospital
PO Box 610
Sheffield, AL 35660
Phone: 256-386-4191
Fax: 256-386-4192
E-mail: **sleep@helenkeller.com**

Tuscaloosa

Snow Sleep Center, PC
701 University Boulevard East
Suite 707
Tuscaloosa, AL 35401
Phone: 205-349-4043
Fax: 205-758-5132

Alaska

Anchorage

Sleep Disorders Center
Providence Alaska Medical Center
3200 Providence Drive
PO Box 196604
Anchorage, AK 99519-6604
Phone: 907-261-3650
Fax: 907-261-4810
E-mail: **JTrodden@provak.org**

Arizona

Glendale

Banner Regional Sleep Disorders
Program
Thunderbird Samaritan Medical Center
in Glendale
5605 West Eugie Avemie
Glendale, AZ 85304
Phone: 602-588-4800
Fax: 602-588-4810
Web Site: bannerhealthaz.com/services/
sleep/sleep.html

Mesa

Banner Regional Sleep Disorders
Program
Desert Samaritan Medical Center
1400 South Dobson Road

Mesa, AZ 85202
Phone: 480-512-3684
Fax: 480-512-8788
Web Site: bannerhealthaz.com/services/
sleep/sleep.html

Phoenix

Banner Regional Sleep Disorders
Program
Good Samaritan Regional Medical
Center
1111 East McDcwell Road
Phoenix, AZ 85006
Phone: 602-239-3990
Fax: 602-239-2129
Web Site: bannerhealthaz.com/services/
sleep/sleep.html

Scottsdale

Sleep Disorders Center at Scottsdale
Healthcare
Scottsdale Healthcare Shea
9003 East Shea Boulevard
Scottsdale, AZ 85260
Phone: 480-860-3200
Fax: 480-860-3251

Tucson

Sleep Disorders Center
University of Arizona
1501 North Campbell Avenue
Tucson, AZ 85724
Phone: 520-694-6112 or 520-626-
6115
Fax: 520-694-2515
E-mail: **squan@resp-sci.arizona.edu**

Yuma

Sleep Center of Yuma
2475 South Avenue A
Suite D
Yuma, AZ 88364
Phone: 928-726-7106
Fax: 928-726-6306
E-mail: **SOA@sleepcenterofyuma.com**
Web Site:
www.sleepcenterofyuma.com

Arkansas

Fayetteville

Sleep Disorders Center
Washington Regional Medical Center
1125 North College Avenue
Fayetteville, AR 72703
Phone: 479-713-1272
Fax: 479-713-1190

Little Rock

St. Vincent Sleep Disorder Center
St. Vincent Health System
#2 St. Vincent Circle
Little Rock, AR 72205
Phone: 501-552-4911
Fax: 501-552-8660
E-mail: **vwofford@stvincenthealth.com**

Little Rock

Arkansas Center for Sleep Medicine
Doctors Building, Suite 506
500 South University Avenue
Little Rock, AR 72205
Phone: 501-661-9191
Fax: 501-661-1991
E-mail: **ARCSMLLC@aol.com**
Web Site: **www.ARSLEEP.COM**

Little Rock

Sleep Disorders Center
Baptist Health Medical Center
9601 I-630, Exit 7
Little Rock, AR 72205-7299
Phone: 501-202-1902
Fax: 501-202-1874
E-mail: **dgdavila@baptist-health.org**
Web Site: **www.baptist-health.com**

Little Rock

pediatric sleep disorders
arkansas children's hospital
800 marshall street
little rock, ar 72202-3591
phone: 501-320-1893
fax: 501-320-6878
e-mail: **rhodeslk@archildrens.org**

California

Anaheim

southern california sleep disorders
specialists
1101 south anaheim boulevard
anaheim, ca 92805
phone: 714-491-1159
fax: 714-563-2865
e-mail: **labbot@uwmc.com**
web site:
www.westernmedanaheim.com

Apple Valley

High Desert Sleep Disorder Center
16017 Tuscola Road
Suite C
Apple Valley, CA 92307
Phone: 760-242-1886
Fax: 760-242-3923

Carmichael

Mercy Sleep Center
6401 Coyle Avenue
Suite 109
Carmichael, CA 95608
Phone: 916-864-5874
Fax: 916-864-5870
E-mail: **rstackmd@chw.edu**
Web Site: **www.pulmonary.org**

Cupertino

Clinical Monitoring Center, Inc.
Sleep Disorders Center
20410 Town Center Lane
Suite F-150
Cupertino, CA 95014
Phone: 408-864-0660
Fax: 408-864-0663
E-mail: **laughtonm@hotmail.com**
Web Site: **www.sleepscape.com**

Fullerton

Sleep Disorders Institute
St. Jude Medical Center
1915 Sunny Crest Drive
Fullerton, CA 92835
Phone: 714-446-7240
Fax: 714-446-7245

Glendale

Glendale Adventist Medical Center
Sleep Disorders Center
Glendale Adventist Medical Center
1509 Wilson Terrace
Glendale, CA 91206
Phone: 818-409-8323
Fax: 818-546-5625
E-mail:
CAVANDKD@GAMCPO.AH.ORG

La Jolla

Pacific Sleep Medicine
9834 Genesee Avenue
Suite 328
La Jolla, CA 92037
Phone: 858-657-0550
Fax: 858-657-0559
E-mail:
sjmsleepmed@compuserve.com
Web Site: **www.sleepmedservices.com**

La Mesa

Sleep Disorders Center
Grossmont Hospital
PO Box 158
La Mesa, CA 91944-0158
Phone: 619-644-4488
Fax: 619-644-402_

Loma Linda

Loma Linda Sleep Disorders Center
Loma Linda University Community
Medical Center
25333 Barton Road
Loma Linda, CA 92354
Phone: 909-558-6344
Fax: 909-558-6343
Web Site: **www.llu.edu/llumc/sleep**

Long Beach

MemorialCare Sleep Disorders Center
Long Beach Memorial Medical Center
2651 Elm Avenue
Suite 307
Long Beach, CA 90806
Phone: 877-536-3314 or 562-424-
6480
Fax: 562-424-1271
Web Site: **www.Memorialcare.com**

Merced

Mercy Medical Center Sleep
Laboratory*
Mercy Medical Center Merced,
Dominican Campus
2740 M Street
Merced, CA 95340
Phone: 209-384-4726
Fax: 209-384-4727
E-mail: **jhoffknecht@CHW.edu**

Mission Viejo

Sleep Disorders Institute
27800 Medical Center Road
Suite 210
Mission Viejo, CA 92691
Phone: 949-347-7400
Fax: 714-446-7245

Monterey

Sleep Disorders Center
Community Hospital of the Monterey
Peninsula
880 Cass Street
Suite 106
Monterey, CA 93940
Phone: 831-641-0136
Fax: 831-641-0149
E-mail: **Sleepcenter@CHOMP.org**

Newport Beach

Sleep Disorders Center
Hoag Memorial Hospital Presbyterian
One Hoag Drive
PO Box 6100
Newport Beach, CA 92658-6100
Phone: 949-760-2070
Fax: 949-574-6297

E-mail: **sleepcenter@hoaghospital.org**
Web Site: **www.hoaghospital.org**

Northridge

Sleep Evaluation Center
Northridge Hospital Medical Center
18300 Roscoe Boulevard
Northridge, CA 91328
Phone: 818-885-5344

Oakland

California Center for Sleep Disorders
3012 Summit Street
5th Floor, South Building
Oakland, CA 94609
Phone: 510-834-8333
Fax: 510-834-4728
E-mail: **sleepsmart@yahoo.com**
Web Site: **www.sleepsmart.com**

Orange

St. Joseph Hospital Sleep Disorders
Center
1310 West Stewart Drive
Suite 403
Orange, CA 92868
Phone: 714-771-8950
Fax: 714-744-8541
Web Site: **SJHSleepCenter.com**

Oxnard

Premier Diagnostics, Inc.
1851 Holser Walk
Suite 210
Oxnard, CA 93030
Phone: 805-485-2633
Fax: 805-485-6650
Web Site: **www.sleep-diagnostics.com**

Pasadena

Sleep Disorders Center
Huntington Memorial Hospital
100 West California Boulevard
PO Box 7013
Pasadena, CA 91109-7013
Phone: 626-397-3061
Fax: 626-397-2194
E-mail: **lucila.gonzalez@schs.com**

Pinole

Sleep Disorders Center
Doctors Medical Center—Pinole
2151 Appian Way
Pinole, CA 94564-2578
Phone: 510-741-2525 or 800-640-9440
Fax: 510-724-2189
E-mail:
GEOFFREY.HUX@tenethealth.com
Web Site: **www.tenethealth.com**

Pomona

Sleep Disorders Center
Pomona Valley Hospital Medical
Center
1798 North Garey Avenue
Pomona, CA 91767
Phone: 909-865-9587
Fax: 909-865-9969
Web Site: **www.PVHMC.org**

Redding

Center for Sleep Disorders of Northern
California
Redding Medical Center
2701 Old Eureka Way
Suite 1I
Redding, CA 96001

Phone: 530-242-6821
Fax: 530-242-6421

Redwood City

Sequoia Sleep Disorders Center
Sequoia Health Services
170 Alameda de las Pulgas
Redwood City, CA 94062-2799
Phone: 650-367-5137
Fax: 650-363-5304
E-mail: **sleep@sleepscene.com**
Web Site: **www.sleepscene.com**

Sacramento

UCDMC Sleep Disorders Center
University of California Davis Medical
Center
2315 Stockton Boulevard
Room 5305
Sacramento, CA 95817
Phone: 916-734-0256
Fax: 916-736-2976

Sacramento

Sutter Sleep Disorders Center
650 Howe Avenue
Suite 910
Sacramento, CA 95825
Phone: 916-646-3300
Fax: 916-646-4603
E-mail: **GROZAD@SutterHealth.org**

San Bernardino

Inland Sleep Center
401 East Highland Avenue
Suite 552
San Bernardino, CA 92404
Phone: 909-883-8058
Fax: 909-881-4607

San Diego

San Diego Sleep Disorders Center
1842 Third Avenue
San Diego, CA 92101
Phone: 619-235-0248
Fax: 619-544-0588
E-mail: **shafor@znet.com**

San Diego

Sleep Disorders Center
Scripps Mercy Hospital
4077 Fifth Avenue
San Diego, CA 92103-2180
Phone: 619-260-7378
Fax: 619-686-3990
Web Site: **www.scrippshealth.org**

San Francisco

Sleep Disorders Center at Mount Zion
University of California, San Francisco
1600 Divisadero Street
San Francisco, CA 94115
Phone: 415-885-7886
Fax: 415-885-3650
E-mail:
Kimberly.Trotter@ucsfmedctr.org
Web Site:
**mountzion.ucsfmedicalcenter.org/
sleep_center/**

Santa Barbara

The Sleep Disorders Center of Santa
Barbara
2410 Fletcher Avenue, Suite 202
Santa Barbara, CA 93105
Phone: 805-898-8845
Fax: 805-898-8848

Santa Monica

Sleep Disorders Center
Santa Monica/UCLA Medical Center
Room 6128
1250 16th Street
Santa Monica, CA 90402
Phone: 310-319-4062
Fax: 310-319-4065

Santa Monica

St. John's Medical Plaza Sleep Disorders
Center
1301 20th Street, Suite 370
Santa Monica, CA 90404
Phone: 310-828-2293
Fax: 310-315-0339
E-mail: **phaberma@ucla.edu**
Web Site: **www.stjohnsleep.com**

Santa Rosa

North Bay Sleep Medicine Institute,
Inc.
2455 Bennett Valley Road
Santa Rosa, CA 95404
Phone: 707-525-9616
Fax: 707-525-0658
E-mail: **nbsmi@nbsmi.com**

Stanford

Sleep Disorders Clinic
Stanford University Medical Center
401 Quarry Road
Suite 3301-A
Stanford, CA 94305
Phone: 650-723-6601
Fax: 650-725-8910
Web Site: **www.stanfordhospital.com**

Stockton

pacific sleep disorders center
3024 pacific avenue
stockton, ca 95204
phone: 209-465-1926 or 209-465-5731
fax: 209-465-0230
e-mail: **psdcstknca@aol.com**
web site: **www.pacificsleepcenter.com**

Thousand Oaks

Southern California Pulmonary and
Sleep Disorders Medical Center
2230 Lynn Road, Suite 101
Thousand Oaks, CA 91360
Phone: 805-557-9930
Fax: 805-557-9940
E-mail: **dontsmoke@earthlink.net**

Torrance

Torrance Memorial Medical Center
Sleep Disorders Center
3330 West Lomita Boulevard
Torrance, CA 90505
Phone: 310-517-4617
Fax: 310-784-4869
Web Site: **www.torrancememorial.org**
and **www.TC4S.com**

Visalia

Sleep Disorders Laboratory*
Kaweah Delta District Hospital
400 West Mineral King Avenue
Visalia, CA 93291
Phone: 559-624-2338
Fax: 559-635-4088
E-mail: **dakins@kdhcd.org**
Web Site: **www.kdhcd.org**

West Hills

West Valley Sleep Disorders Center
7320 Woodlake Avenue, Suite 140
West Hills, CA 91307
Phone: 818-715-0096
Fax: 818-716-1875
E-mail: **gordon@dowds.com**

Woodland

Sleep Disorders Center
Woodland Memorial Hospital
1325 Cottonwood Street
Woodland, CA 95695
Phone: 530-669-5555
Fax: 530-662-9174
E-mail: **cmacias@chw.edu**

Colorado

Colorado Springs

Memorial Sleep Disorders Center
Memorial Hospital
1400 E. Boulder Street
Colorado Springs, CO 80909
Phone: 719-365-5075
Fax: 791-365-6808
E-mail: **carrie.tyler@memhospcs.org**

Denver

The Sleep Center at National Jewish
Medical Center
1400 Jackson Street, A200
Denver, CO 80206
Phone: 303-270-2708
Fax: 303-270-2109
E-mail: **BallardR@NJC.org**
Web Site: **www.nationaljewish.org**

Loveland

Sleep Disorders Centers of Northern
Colorado
Mike Medical Center
2000 N. Boise Avenue
Loveland, CO 80539-0830
Phone: 970-635-4027
Fax: 970-593-6040

Pueblo

Sleep Center of Southern Colorado
Parkview Medical Center
400 West 16th Street
Pueblo, CO 81003
Phone: 719-584-4976
Fax: 719-584-4929
E-mail:
george_juszynski@parkviewmc.com
Web Site: www.parkviewmc.com/
sleep.htm

Wheat Ridge

Wheat Ridge
Sleep Disorders Laboratory
Exempla Lutheran Medical Center
8300 West 38th Avenue
Wheat Ridge, CO 80033
Phone: 303-425-8574
Fax: 303-403-3665

Connecticut

Danbury

Danbury Hospital Sleep Disorders
Center
Danbury Hospital
24 Hospital Avenue
Danbury, CT 06810
Phone: 203-731-8033

Fax: 203-731-8628
E-mail: Kotcha@DanHosp.org

Fairfield

Gaylord/Fairfield Sleep Services
1495 Black Rock Turnpike
Fairfield, CT 06430
Phone: 203-624-3140
Fax: 203-495-8569
E-mail: dclark@gaylord.org
Web Site: www.gaylord.org

Greenwich

The Sleep Laboratory at Greenwich
Hospital*
Greenwich Hospital
5 Perryridge Road
Greenwich, CT 06830
Phone: 203-863-3167
Fax: 203-863-3996
E-mail: DaveP@greenhosp.chime.org
Web Site: www.greenhosp.org/
medicalservices_sleep.asp

Manchester

Sleep Disorders Laboratory*
Manchester Memorial Hospital
71 Haynes Street
Manchester, CT 06040
Phone: 860-647-6881
Fax: 860-533-2943
E-mail: TFarrell@MMHosp.chime.org
Web Site: www.echn.org/sleeplab.htm

New Britain

Sleep Disorders Center
New Britain General Hospital
100 Grand Street
New Britain, CT 06050-0100

Phone: 860-224-5538
Fax: 860-224-5739
Web Site: **www.nbgh.org/sleep.html**

New Haven

Gaylord/New Haven Sleep Services
One Long Wharf Drive
New Haven, CT 06511
Phone: 203-624-3140
Fax: 203-495-8569
E-mail: **dclark@gaylord.org**
Web Site: **www.gaylord.org**

New Haven

Yale Center for Sleep Medicine
Yale University School of Medicine
40 Temple Street
Suite 3C
New Haven, CT 06510
Phone: 203-764-6788
Fax: 203-764-6787
E-mail: **sleep.disorders@yale.edu**
Web Site: **www.info.med.yale.edu/
intmed/sleep**

New London

Gaylord/New London Sleep Services
470 Bank Street
New London, CT 06320
Phone: 203-624-3140
Fax: 203-495-8569
E-mail: **dclark@gaylord.org**
Web Site: **www.gaylord.org**

Norwalk

The Sleep Disorders Center
Norwalk Hospital
Maple Street
Norwalk, CT 06856

Phone: 203-855-3632
Fax: 203-852-2945
E-mail:
ed.o'malley@norwalkhealth.org
Web Site: **www.norwalkhosp.org**

Norwich

Yale Center for Sleep Medicine/Eastern
Connecticut
Yale University
1 Towne Park Plaza
Norwich, CT 06360
Phone: 877-925-3736
Fax: 860-823-1896
E-mail: **sleep.disorders@yale.edu**
Web Site: **www.info.med.yale.edu/
intmed/sleep/**

Wallingford

Gaylord/Wallingford Sleep Disorders
Laboratory*
Gaylord Hospital Inc.
PO Box 400
Gaylord Farm Road
Wallingford, CT 06492
Phone: 203-284-2853
Fax: 203-284-2746
E-mail: **cpolaske@gaylord.org**
Web Site: **www.gaylord.org**

West Hartford

Gaylord/West Hartford Sleep Services
836 Farmington Avenue
West Hartford, CT 06119
Phone: 203-624-3140
Fax: 203-495-8569
E-mail: **cpolaske@gaylord.org**
Web Site: **www.gaylord.org**

Willimantic

Windham Hospital Diagnostic Sleep
Laboratory*
Windham Community Memorial
Hospital
112 Mansfield Avenue
Willimantic, CT 06226
Phone: 860-456-6853
Fax: 860-456-6890
E-mail: **jflood@wcmh.org**
Web Site: **www.windhamhospital.org**

Delaware

Newark

Sleep Disorders Center
Christiana Care Health Services
4755 Ogletown-Stanton Road
PO Box 6001
Newark, DE 19718
Phone: 302-428-4600
Fax: 302-733-2533
E-mail: **mhancock@christianacare.org**

Wilmington

Sleep Disorders Center
Christiana Care Health Services
Wilmington Hospital
501 West 14th Street
Wilmington, DE 19899
Phone: 302-428-4600
Fax: 302-733-2533
E-mail: **mhancock@christianacare.org**

District of Columbia

Washington

Sleep Disorders Center, 5 Main
Hospital

Georgetown University Hospital
3800 Reservoir Road NW
Washington, DC 20007-2197
Phone: 202-784-3610
Fax: 202-784-2920
E-mail:
knightk@gunet.georgetown.edu

Washington

Sibley Memorial Hospital Sleep
Disorders Center
5255 Loughboro Road NW
Washington, DC 20016
Phone: 202-364-7676
Fax: 202-362-9378

Florida

Boca Raton

Boca Raton Sleep Disorders Center
660 Glades Road, Building C
Suite 220
Boca Raton, FL 33486
Phone: 561-750-9881
Fax: 561-750-9644
E-mail: **bocasleep@aol.com**

Celebration

Florida Hospital Celebration Health
Florida Hospital
400 Celebration Place
Celebration, FL 34747
Phone: 407-303-4002
Fax: 407-303-4303

Fort Lauderdale

Sleep Disorders Center
Broward General Medical Center
1600 South Andrews Avenue

Fort Lauderdale, FL 33316
Phone: 954-355-5532
Fax: 954-468-8092
E-mail: **RLETOILE@NBHD.ORG**

Jacksonville

Mayo Sleep Disorders Center
Mayo Clinic Jacksonville
4500 San Pablo Road
Jacksonville, FL 32224
Phone: 904-953-7287
Fax: 904-953-7388

Lakeland

Watson Clinic Sleep Disorders Center
The Watson Clinic, LLP
1600 Lakeland Hills Boulevard
PO Box 95000
Lakeland, FL 33804-5000
Phone: 941-680-7627
Fax: 941-680-7430

Melbourne

Atlantic Sleep Disorders Center
1401 South Apollo Boulevard, Suite A
Melbourne, FL 32901
Phone: 321-952-5191
Fax: 321-952-7262
E-mail: **Atlantic.Sleep@aol.com**
Web Site: **doctor.medscape.com/
DennisKingMD**

Miami

University of Miami School of
Medicine
JMH and VA Medical Center Sleep
Disorders Center
Department of Neurology
P.O. Box 016960

Miami, FL 33101
Phone: 305-243-5195

Miami

Sleep Disorders Center
Miami Children's Hospital
6125 Southwest 31st Street
Miami, FL 33155
Phone: 305-669-7136
Fax: 305-669-6472
E-mail: **Maderay@aol.com**

Miami

Mercy Hospital
3663 South Miami Avenue, Suite 5510
Miami, FL 33133
Phone: 305-860-5208
Fax: 305-285-5075
E-mail: **slp0002@mercymiami.org**

Miami Beach

Sleep Disorders Center
Mt. Sinai Medical Center
4300 Alton Road
Miami Beach, FL 33140
Phone: 305-674-2613
Fax: 305-674-2647

Orlando

Florida Hospital Sleep Disorders Center
601 East Rollins Avenue
Orlando, FL 32803
Phone: 407-303-1558
Fax: 407-303-1775
E-mail: **Patricia_Zable@mail.fhms.net**

Orlando

Orlando Sleep Disorders Center
1118 South Orange Avenue, Suite 102
Orlando, FL 32806
Phone: 407-649-6869
Fax: 407-872-3876
E-mail: **orlsleep@bellsouth.net**

Palm Bay

Health First Sleep Disorders Center
Palm Bay Community Hospital
1425 Malabar Road NE, Suite 250
Palm Bay, FL 32907
Phone: 321-434-8087
Fax: 321-434-8496
E-mail: **Coreen.Downey@health-first.org**
Web Site: **health-first.org/hospitals_services/pbch/sleep_center.cfm**

Pensacola

Sleep Disorders Center
West Florida Hospital
8383 North Davis Highway
Pensacola, FL 32514
Phone: 850-494-4850
Fax: 850-494-4809
Web Site: **westfloridahospital.com**

Pensacola

Baptist Hospital Sleep Disorders Center
Baptist Hospital
1000 West Moreno Street
Pensacola, FL 32501
Phone: 850-469-7042
Fax: 850-469-2263
E-mail: **njenkins@bhcpens.org**

Pompano Beach

Sleep Disorders Center
North Broward Medical Center
201 East Sample Road
Pompano Beach, FL 33064
Phone: 954-786-7399
Fax: 954-786-7342

Punta Gorda

Sleep Disorders Center
Charlotte Regional Medical Center
733 East Olympia Avenue
Punta Gorda, FL 33950
Phone: 941-637-3141
Fax: 941-637-3189
E-mail: **jlewis@crmc.hma_corp.com**

Sarasota

Sleep Disorders Center
Sarasota Memorial Hospital
1700 South Tamiami Trail
Sarasota, FL 34239
Phone: 941-917-2525
Fax: 941-917-6187
E-mail: **SLEEP-LAB@SMH.COM**

St. Petersburg

St. Petersburg Sleep Disorders Center
Palms of Pasadena Hospital
1501 Pasadena Avenue South
St. Petersburg, FL 33707
Phone: 727-360-0853 or 800-242-3244
(in Florida)

Tallahassee

Tallahassee Sleep Disorders Center
2013 Miccosukee Road

Tallahassee, FL 32308
Phone: 800-662-4278 x4 or 850-878-7271
Fax: 850-878-1509
E-mail: N47593@aol.com

Tampa

The Sleep Center
University Community Hospital
3100 East Fletcher Avenue
Tampa, FL 33613
Phone: 813-615-7410
Fax: 813-615-0878
E-mail:
thetampasleepcenter@yahoo.com
Web Site: www.uch.org

Georgia

Atlanta

Sleep Disorders Center of Georgia
5505 Peachtree Dunwoody Road, Suite 380
Atlanta, GA 30342
Phone: 404-257-0080
Fax: 404-257-0592
E-mail: alanl@sleepsciences.com
Web Site: sleepsciences.com

Atlanta

Sleep Disorders Center
Northside Hospital
5780 Peachtree Dunwoody Road, Suite 150
Atlanta, GA 30342
Phone: 404-851-8135
Fax: 404-252-9946
E-mail: nshsleep@mindspring.com
Web Site: www.nshsleep.com

Atlanta

APG Center for Sleep Disorders
5667 Peachtree Dunwoody Road, Suite 250
Atlanta, GA 30342
Phone: 404-851-6688
Fax: 404-851-6604
E-mail:
DWESTERMAN@SJHA.ORG

Atlanta

Atlanta Center for Sleep Disorders
Box 44
303 Parkway Drive
Atlanta, GA 30312
Phone: 404-265-3722
Fax: 404-265-3833
E-mail: robert.speers@tenethealth.com
Web Site: www.atlantamedcenter.com

Atlanta

Sleep Disorders Center
Children's Healthcare of Atlanta
1600 Tullie Circle
Atlanta, GA 30329
Phone: 404-250-2096
Fax: 404-257-3291
E-mail: Lesa.Kervin@CHOA.org

Atlanta

The Sleep Center at Piedmont Hospital
1968 Peachtree Road NW
Atlanta, GA 30309
Phone: 404-605-4278
Fax: 404-367-3594
E-mail:
Osterman_Shelia@Piedmont.Promina.org
Web Site: www.piedmonthospital.org

Decatur

Sleep Disorder Center
DeKalb Medical Center
2665 North Decatur Road, Suite 435
Decatur, GA 30033
Phone: 404-501-5927
Fax: 404-501-7088

Macon

SleepMed of Central Georgia
770 Hemlock Street
PO Box 1035
Macon, GA 31202
Phone: 478-745-9050
Fax: 478-745-5125
E-mail: cjackson@sleepmed_md
Web Site: www.sleepmed.md

Marietta

WellStar Sleep Disorders Center
Windy Hill Hospital
2540 Windy Hill Road
Marietta, GA 30067
Phone: 770-644-1755
Fax: 770-644-1759
E-mail: Keller_Susan@Wellstar.org

Riverdale

The Sleep Disorder Centers of
Southeastern Lung Care in South
Atlanta
181 Upper Riverdale Road
Building A, Suite 2
Riverdale, GA 30296
Phone: 770-994-3008
Fax: 770-994-3883

Rome

Sleep Disorders Center
Redmond Regional Medical Center
501 Redmond Road
Rome, GA 30165
Phone: 706-802-3955
Fax: 706-802-3957
E-mail:
Angie.Riddle@HCAHealthcare.com
Web Site: www.Redmondregional.com

Savannah

Savannah Sleep Disorders Center
at Saint Joseph's Hospital
#1 St. Joseph's Professional Plaza
11706 Mercy Boulevard
Savannah, GA 31419
Phone: 912-927-5141
Fax: 912-921-3380
E-mail: yawn@drsleepwell.com
Web Site: www.sleepcor.com

Savannah

Sleep Disorders Center
Memorial Health University Medical
Center
4700 Waters Avenue
Savannah, GA 31403
Phone: 912-350-8327
Fax: 912-350-7281

Savannah

Department of Sleep Disorders
Medicine
Candler Hospital
5353 Reynolds Street
Savannah, GA 31405
Phone: 912-692-6673
Fax: 912-692-6931

E-mail: **RockettP@stjosephs-candler.org**
Web Site: **www.stjosephs-candler.org**

Hawaii

Honolulu

Sleep Disorders Center of the Pacific
Straub Clinic & Hospital
888 South King Street
Honolulu, HI 96813
Phone: 808-522-4448
Fax: 808-522-3048
E-mail: **lkapuniai@straub.net**
lkapuniai@straub.
net lkapuniai@straub.net

Honolulu

Hawaii Center for Sleep Medicine,
LTD.
2130 South Beretania Street
Honolulu, HI 96826
Phone: 808-944-8464

Honolulu

Queen's Medical Center Sleep
Laboratory*
The Queen's Medical Center
1301 Punchbowl Street
Honolulu, HI 96813
Phone: 808-547-4396
Fax: 808-537-7830
E-mail: **cagard@queens.org**

Kihei

Maui Chest Medicine
380 Huku Lii Place
Kihei, HI 96753

Phone: 808-874-8774
Fax: 808-874-8947

Idaho

Boise

Idaho Sleep Disorders Center
St. Luke's Regional Medical
Center—Boise
190 East Bannock Street
Boise, ID 83712
Phone: 208-381-2440 and 208-706-5380
Fax: 208-381-4341
E-mail: **GABLEM@SLRMC.ORG**

Lewiston

SJRMC Sleep Lab
St. Joseph Regional Medical Center
415 Sixth Street
Lewiston, ID 83501
Phone: 208-799-5484
Fax: 208-799-5789

Nampa

Idaho Sleep Disorders Center-Nampa
Mercy Medical Center
1512 12th Avenue Road
Nampa, ID 83686
Phone: 208-463-5082
Fax: 208-463-5087

Twin Falls

Idaho Diagnostic Sleep Lab*
526-C Shoup Avenue West
Twin Falls, ID 83301
Phone: 208-736-7646
Fax: 208-736-1569
E-mail: **Info@Idsleeplab.com**

Illinois

Belleville

Southern Illinois Sleep Disorders
Center
St. Elizabeth's Hospital
211 South Third Street
Belleville, IL 62220
Phone: 888-650-7474
Fax: 618-222-4660
E-mail: **SDASHNER@SEBH.ORG**

Chicago

Sleep Disorders Center
The University of Chicago Hospitals
5841 South Maryland
MC2091
Chicago, IL 60637
Phone: 773-702-1782
Fax: 773-702-7998
E-mail:
jpspire@neurology.bsd.uchicago.edu

Chicago

Sleep Disorder Service and Research
Center
Rush-Presbyterian-St. Luke's Medical
Center
1653 West Congress Parkway
Chicago, IL 60612
Phone: 312-942-5440
Fax: 312-942-8961
E-mail: **estepans@rush.edu**
Web Site: **www.rush.edu/Med/Psych/
sleep.html**

Chicago

Sleep Disorders Center
Northwestern Memorial Hospital

201 East Huron, Galter 7th Floor
Chicago, IL 60611
Phone: 312-926-2650
Fax: 312-926-6637
E-mail: **p-zee@nwu.edu**
Web Site: **www.nmh.org**

Chicago

Center for Sleep and Ventilatory
Disorders
University of Illinois at Chicago
M/C 722
1740 West Taylor Street—Room 536E
Chicago, IL 60612
Phone: 312-996-7708
Fax: 312-413-0503
E-mail: **dsewitch@uic.edu**

Chicago

Sleep Medicine Center
Children's Memorial Hospital
2300 Children's Plaza, Box 43
Chicago, IL 60614-3394
Phone: 773-880-8230
Fax: 773-880-6300
E-mail: **ssheldon@northwestern.edu**

Des Plaines

Holy Family Sleep Disorders Center
Holy Family Medical Center
100 North River Road
Des Plaines, IL 60016
Phone: 847-297-1800ext. 2080
Fax: 847-813-3007

Elk Grove Village

Sleep Disorders Center
Alexian Brothers Medical Center
810 Biesterfield Road, Suite 409

Elk Grove Village, IL 60007
Phone: 847-981-5926
Fax: 847-981-2003

Evanston

Sleep Disorders Center
Evanston Hospital
2650 Ridge Avenue
Evanston, IL 60201
Phone: 847-570-2567
Fax: 847-570-2984
E-mail: **rrosenberg@enh.org**

Hinsdale

Sleep Disorders Center
Hinsdale Hospital
120 North Oak Street
Hinsdale, IL 60521
Phone: 630-655-4803
Fax: 630-655-8166
E-mail: **Rpolak@ahssorg.com**
Web Site: **www.ahsmidwest.org**

Mattoon

Carle Regional Sleep Disorders Center/
Mattoon Branch
Carle Clinic
200 Lerna Road South
Mattoon, IL 61938
Phone: 217-383-3198
Fax: 217-383-7117
E-mail: **sleep.lab@carle.com**

Oak Park

West Suburban Snoring & Sleep
Disorders Center
West Suburban Health Care
One Erie Court, Suite 3000
Oak Park, IL 60302

Phone: 708-383-9928
Fax: 708-383-1619

Orland Park

The Center for Sleep Medicine
9631 West 153rd Street, Suite 38
Orland Park, IL 60462
Phone: 708-364-0261
Fax: 708-364-0259
E-mail:
AMOUTON@Sleepmedcenter.com

Park Ridge

Sleep Disorders Center
Lutheran General Hospital
1775 Dempster Street
Parkside Center, Suite B06
Park Ridge, IL 60068
Phone: 847-723-7024
Fax: 847-723-7369
E-mail:
**BARRY.WEBER@ADVOCATEMED
ICAL.COM**

Peoria

C. Duane Morgan Sleep Disorders
Center
Methodist Medical Center of Illinois
221 Northeast Glen Oak Avenue
Peoria, IL 61636
Phone: 309-672-4966
Fax: 309-672-4117
E-mail: **rwizieck@mmci.org**
Web Site: **www.mmci.org**

Skokie

Sleep & Behavior Medicine Institute at
RNSMC
9700 North Kenton Avenue, Suite K-

205
Skokie, IL 60076
Phone: 847-673-8005
Fax: 847-673-8719
E-mail: **golbina@aol.com**

Springfield

SIU School of Medicine/Memorial
Medical Center
Sleep Disorders Center
Memorial Medical Center
701 North First
Springfield, IL 62781
Phone: 217-788-4269
Fax: 217-788-7057
E-mail: **jhenkle@siumed.edu**

Sterling

CGH Sleep Center
CGH Medical Center
100 East Le Feure Road
Sterling, IL 61081
Phone: 815-625-0400 ext. 5687
Fax: 815-625-0203
E-mail: **sleepcenter@chguic.com**

Urbana

Carle Regional Sleep Disorders Center
Carle Foundation Hospital
611 West Park Street
Urbana, IL 61801-2595
Phone: 217-383-3364
Fax: 217-383-7117
E-mail: **sleep.lab@carle.com**

Winfield

Center for Sleep Health
Central Du Page Hospital
Robert McCormick Pavilion, Entrance

E, 3rd Floor
25 North Winfield Road
Winfield, IL 60190
Phone: 630-933-2975
Fax: 630-933-2745

Indiana

Beech Grove

Sleep Disorders Center
St. Francis Hospital and Health Centers
1500 Albany Street, Suite 1110
Beech Grove, IN 46107
Phone: 317-783-8144
Fax: 317-781-1402

Corydon

Harrison County Hospital Center for
Sleep Disorders
Harrison County Hospital
245 Atwood Street
Corydon, IN 47112
Phone: 812-738-7889
Fax: 812-738-7853
E-mail: **kkeigher@harrisoncohosp.org**

Evansville

Southwestern Indiana Sleep Disorders
Center
Sleep Medicine Associates, P.C.
445 Cross Pointe Boulevard, Suite 230
Evansville, IN 47715
Phone: 812-473-1737
Fax: 812-473-2432
Web Site:
www.sleepneverfeltsogood.com

Evansville

Sleep Disorders Center
St. Mary's Medical Center
1400 Professional Boulevard, Suite 135
Evansville, IN 47714
Phone: 812-476-5140
Fax: 812-476-5688

Fort Wayne

St. Joseph Sleep Disorders Center
St. Joseph Medical Center
700 Broadway
Fort Wayne, IN 46802
Phone: 260-425-3552
Fax: 219-425-3553

Indianapolis

Sleep Disorders Center
St. Vincent Hospital and Health
Services
8401 Harcourt Road
Indianapolis, IN 46260-0160
Phone: 317-338-2152
Fax: 317-338-4917
E-mail: **sleepctr@stvincent.org**
Web Site: **www.stvincent.org**

Indianapolis

Methodist Sleep Disorders Center
Clarian Health
I-65 at 21st Street, P. O. Box 1367
Indianapolis, IN 46206-1367
Phone: 317-962-5706
Fax: 317-962-8703
E-mail: **TEhle@clarian.com**

Indianapolis

Sleep/Wake Disorders Center
Community Hospitals Indianapolis
1500 North Ritter Avenue
Indianapolis, IN 46219
Phone: 317-355-4275
Fax: 317-351-2785
E-mail: **MEVOLLMER@POL.NET**

Indianapolis

Sleep/Wake Disorders Center
Winona Memorial Hospital
3232 North Meridian Street
Indianapolis, IN 46208
Phone: 317-927-2100
Fax: 317-927-2914

Indianapolis

Center for Sleep Disorders
Indiana University School of Medicine
550 North University Boulevard/
UH5450
Indianapolis, IN 46202
Phone: 317-274-2136 or 317-274-
0943
Fax: 317-274-4224
E-mail: **sleeplab@iupui.edu**
Web Site: **medicine.iupui.edu/sleeplab**

Lafayette

Sleep Disorder Center
St. Elizabeth Medical Center
1501 Hartford Street
Lafayette, IN 47904
Phone: 765-423-6518
Fax: 765-423-6525

New Albany

Floyd Memorial Hospital Sleep Lab
1850 State Street
New Albany, IN 47150
Phone: 812-949-5550
Fax: 812-949-5748

Iowa

Ames

Sleep Disorders Center
Mary Greeley Medical Center
1111 Duff Avenue
Ames, IA 50010
Phone: 515-239-2353
Fax: 515-239-6741
E-mail: **SleepLab@MGMC.com**
Web Site: **www.MGMC.org**

Davenport

Genesis Sleep Disorders Center
Genesis Medical Center
1227 East Rusholme
Davenport, IA 52803
Phone: 319-421-1523
Fax: 319-421-1539
E-mail: **RasmusS@genesishealth.com**
Web Site: **www.genesishealth.com**

Des Moines

Sleep Center at Mercy
Mercy Medical Center
1111 Sixth Avenue
Des Moines, IA 50314-2611
Phone: 515-247-3171
Fax: 515-643-8905
E-mail: **abarth@mercydesmoines.org**

Iowa City

Sleep Disorders Center
The Department of Neurology
The University of Iowa Hospitals and
Clinics
Iowa City, IA 52242
Phone: 319-356-3813
Fax: 319-356-4505
E-mail: **mark-dyken@uiowa.edu**

Kansas

Hays

Sleep Disorders Center
The Center for Health Improvement
2500 Canterbury Drive
Hays, KS 67601
Phone: 785-623-5373
Fax: 785-623-5377
E-mail: **sbollig@haysmed.com**

Overland Park

Saint Luke's South Sleep Disorders
Center
Saint Luke's Hospital
12300 Metcalf Avenue
Overland Park, KS 66213
Phone: 913-317-7765
Fax: 913-317-7468

Overland Park

Sleep Disorders Center
Overland Park Regional Medical
Center
10500 Quivira Road
PO Box 15959
Overland Park, KS 66215
Phone: 913-541-5641
Fax: 913-541-5443

E-mail:
mianderson@healthmidwest.org
Web Site: www.healthmidwest.org/
respiratory

Shawnee Mission

Sleep Lab at Shawnee Mission Medical
Center
Shawnee Mission Medical Center
9100 W 74th Street
Shawnee Mission, KS 66204
Phone: 913-676-8112
Fax: 913-789-3914

Topeka

Sleep Disorders Center
St. Francis Hospital and Medical
Center
1700 Southwest Seventh Street
Topeka, KS 66606-1690
Phone: 785-295-7900
Fax: 785-231-5979
E-mail:
david.miller@stfrancistopeka.org

Wichita

Sleep Medicine Center of Kansas
Wichita Clinic
818 North Carriage Parkway
Wichita, KS 67208
Phone: 316-651-2250
Fax: 316-685-9391
E-mail: Bennettag@wichitaclinic.com
Web Site: www.wichitaclinic.com

Kentucky

Bowling Green

Sleep Disorders Center
Greenview Regional Hospital
1801 Ashley Circle
Bowling Green, KY 42101
Phone: 270-793-2175
Fax: 270-793-2177

Bowling Green

Physicians' Center for Sleep Disorders
Graves-Gilbert Clinic
PO Box 90007
Bowling Green, KY 42102-9007
Phone: 270-781-8420
Fax: 270-781-0565
E-mail: zachekm@Graves-
GilbertClinic.com

Flemingsburg

The Sleep Lab at Fleming County
Hospital*
Fleming County Hospital
920 Elizaville Avenue, P.O. Box 388
Flemingsburg, KY 41041
Phone: 606-849-5029
Fax: 606-849-5184

Florence

Sleep Disorders Center
St. Luke Hospital
7380 Turfway Road
Florence, KY 41042
Phone: 859-962-5347
Fax: 859-572-3375
E-mail: stevenjscheer@usa.net
Web Site: www.drscheer.go.to

Fort Thomas

The Sleep Disorder Center of St. Luke
Hospital
St. Luke Hospital, Inc.
85 North Grand Avenue
Fort Thomas, KY 41075
Phone: 859-572-3535
Fax: 859-572-3375
E-mail: **stevenjscheer@usa.net**
Web Site: **drscheer.go.to**

Frankford

Sleep Medicine Specialists of Frankfort
Sleep Medicine Specialists
1006 Leawood Drive, Suite 100
Frankford, KY 40601
Phone: 502-223-5200
Fax: 502-223-8900

Greenville

MCH Sleep Apnea Center*
Muhlenberg Community Hospital
440 Hopkinsville St.
Greenville, KY 42345
Phone: 270-754-3971
Fax: 270-754-3299

Henderson

Methodist Hospital Sleep Lab*
Methodist Hospital
1305 North Elm Street
Henderson, KY 42420
Phone: 270-827-7474
Fax: 270-827-7371

Hopkinsville

sleep apnea center*
jennie stuart medical center

320 west 18th street
hopkinsville, ky 42240
phone: 270-887-0410
fax: 270-887-0412
e-mail: **mpiercerpsgt@netscape.net**

Lexington

Sleep Center
Samaritan Hospital
310 South Limestone
Lexington, KY 40508
Phone: 859-226-7006
Fax: 859-226-7008
Web Site: **www.KYSS.org** or
SamaritanHospital.org

Lexington

Sleep Disorders Center
St. Joseph's Hospital
One St. Joseph Drive
Lexington, KY 40504
Phone: 859-313-1855
Fax: 859-313-3021
E-mail:
a_kathryn_hansen@SJHLex.org

Louisville

Sleep Medicine Specialists
1169 Eastern Parkway
Suite 3357
Louisville, KY 40217
Phone: 502-454-0755
Fax: 502-454-3497

Louisville

Sleep Disorders Center
Norton Audubon Hospital
One Audubon Plaza Drive
Louisville, KY 40217

Phone: 502-636-7459
Fax: 502-636-7474
E-mail:
sleepisourjob@nortonhealthcare.org
Web Site: **www.nortonhealthcare.com**
or **www.kyss.org**

Louisville

Sleep Disorders Center
University of Louisville Hospital
530 South Jackson Street
Louisville, KY 40202
Phone: 502-562-3792
Fax: 502-562-4632
E-mail: **Barbarig@ULH.org**
Web Site: **www.ulh.org**

Louisville

Sleep Disorders Center
Baptist Hospital East
4002 Kresge Way
Louisville, KY 40207
Phone: 502-896-7612
Fax: 502-897-8238
E-mail: **KGross1@bhsi.COM**

Louisville

Caritas Sleep Disorders Center
Caritas Medical Center
1850 Bluegrass Avenue
Louisville, KY 40215
Phone: 502-361-6555
Fax: 502-361-6554
E-mail: **darleneherps@chi-caritas.org**

Madisonville

Regional Medical Center
Sleep Disorders Lab*
900 Hospital Drive

Madisonville, KY 42431
Phone: 270-825-5918
Fax: 270-825-5159
E-mail: **klouden@trover.org**
Web Site: **troverfoundation.org**

Owensboro

OMHS Sleep Laboratory*
Owensboro Mercy Health System
811 East Parrish
Owensboro, KY 42303
Phone: 270-688-2882 Mr. Sisley or
270-688-5221 Sleep Lab;
Fax: 270-688-2624
E-mail: **msisley@omhs.org**

Paducah

Diller Regional Sleep Disorders Center
Lourdes Hospital
1530 Lone Oak Road
Paducah, KY 42003
Phone: 270-444-2660
Fax: 270-444-2661
E-mail: **Neurodocs@AOL.COM**

Paris

The Sleep Lab*
9 Linville Drive
Paris, KY 40361
Phone: 859-987-1127
Fax: 859-987-5009
E-mail:
Bruce.Carter@LifepointHospitals.com

Pikeville

Sleep Center
Pikeville Methodist Hospital
911 Bypass Road
Pikeville, KY 41501

Phone: 606-437-3989
Fax: 606-437-9649

Richmond

P.A.C. Sleep Disorders Lab*
Pattie A. Clay Hospital
PO Box 1600
801 Eastern Bypass
Richmond, KY 40475
Phone: 859-625-3334
Fax: 859-625-3104

Scottsville

The Medical Center Sleep Center
456 Burnley Road
Scottsville, KY 42164
Phone: 270-622-2865
Fax: 270-622-2949
E-mail: SLEEP@MCBG.ORG
Web Site: www.mcbg.org/scottsville/
sleeplab/default.htm

Somerset

Sleep Disorders Center of LCRH
Lake Cumberland Regional Hospital
305 Langdon Street
Somerset, KY 42503
Phone: 606-678-3414
Fax: 606-678-3419
E-mail:
kevin.gregory@lifepointhospitals.com

Versailles

The Sleep Lab
Bluegrass Community Hospital
360 Amsden Avenue
Versailles, KY 40383
Phone: 859-879-2321
Fax: 859-879-2303

E-mail:
denise.enlow@lifepointhospital.org

Louisiana

Lafayette

Lourdes Sleep Disorders Center
Our Lady of Lourdes Regional Medical
Center
100 Asma Boulevard
Building 1, Suite 205
Lafayette, LA 70508
Phone: 337-289-5605
Fax: 337-289-5609
E-mail: soileauc@lourdesrmc.com
Web Site: www.lourdes.net

Lake Charles

Sleep Disorder Center of Louisiana
4820 Lake Street
Lake Charles, LA 70605
Phone: 337-310-7378
Fax: 337-310-7382
E-mail:
lhornsby@sleepdisordercenterofla.com

New Orleans

Tulane Sleep Disorders Center
1415 Tulane Avenue
Box HC17
New Orleans, LA 70112
Phone: 504-584-1657
Fax: 504-988-4583
E-mail: DRDSHARON@AOL.COM

New Orleans

Memorial Medical Center Sleep
Disorders Center
2700 Napoleon Avenue

New Orleans, LA 70115
Phone: 504-896-5439
Fax: 504-897-4421
E-mail: **gsf0802@aol.com**

Opelousas

Sleep Disorders Center
Opelousas General Hospital
539 East Prudhomme Street
PO Box 1389
Opelousas, LA 70570
Phone: 337-943-7146
Fax: 337-594-3837
E-mail:
sleepcenter@opelousasgeneral.com
Web Site: **www.opelousasgeneral.com**

Shreveport

LSU Sleep Disorders Center
Louisiana State University Health
Sciences Center
PO Box 33932
Shreveport, LA 71130-3932
Phone: 318-675-5365
Fax: 318-675-4440
E-mail: **ACHESS@LSUHSC.EDU**

Shreveport

The Neurology and Sleep Clinic
2205 East 70th Street
Shreveport, LA 71105
Phone: 318-797-1585
Fax: 318-797-6077
E-mail: **Namouf@earthlink.net**

Slidell

Sleep Disorders Center
Slidell Memorial Hospital and Medical
Center

1001 Gause Boulevard
Slidell, LA 70458
Phone: 985-649-8823
Fax: 985-649-8711
E-mail: **mcmanust@smh.plus.org**

Slidell

NorthShore Sleep Disorders Center
NorthShore Regional Medical Center
350 Gateway Drive
Suite A
Slidell, LA 70461
Phone: 504-646-5711
Fax: 504-646-5013
E-mail:
Mary.B.Jones@tenethealth.com

Thibodaux

Thibodaux Regional and Sleep
Disorders Center
602 N. Acadia Road
Thibodaux, LA 70301
Phone: 985-493-4759
Fax: 985-449-2525
E-mail:
sleepstudycenter@thibodaux.com
Web Site: **www.thibodaux.com**

West Monroe

Sleep Apnea Center
Glenwood Regional Medical Center
503 McMillan Road
West Monroe, LA 71291
Phone: 318-329-3662
Fax: 318-329-4866
E-mail: **cphillips@grmc.com**

Maine

Lewiston

St. Mary's Sleep Disorders Center
St. Mary's Regional Medical Center
77 Bates Street
Lewiston, ME 04240
Phone: 207-777-8959
Fax: 207-753-3093

Portland

Maine Sleep Institute
22 Bramhall Street
Portland, ME 04102-3134
Phone: 207-871-4535
Fax: 207-871-6005

Maryland

Baltimore

The Johns Hopkins Sleep Disorders
Center
Asthma and Allergy Building, Room
4B50
Johns Hopkins Bayview Medical Center
5501 Hopkins Bayview Circle
Baltimore, MD 21224
Phone: 410-550-0571
Fax: 410-550-3374
E-mail: **nschuber@maic.jhmi.edu**

Baltimore

The Johns Hopkins Pediatric Sleep
Center
Mt. Washington Pediatric Hospital
1708 West Rogers Avenue
Baltimore, MD 21209
Phone: 410-955-1103
Fax: 410-955-1030

E-mail: **cmarcus@welch.jhu.edu**
Web Site: **www.mwph.org**

Baltimore

The Johns Hopkins Pediatric Sleep
Center
Johns Hopkins Hospital
Park 316
600 North Wolfe Street
Baltimore, MD 21287
Phone: 410-955-1103
Fax: 410-614-9811
E-mail: **ahamer@jhmi.edu**

Easton

Regional Sleep Disorders Center
Memorial Hospital at Easton
219 South Washington Street
Easton, MD 21601
Phone: 410-822-1000 x5338
Fax: 410-820-7831
E-mail: **gpoole@shorehealth.org**

Hagerstown

The Sleep-Breathing Disorders Center
of Hagerstown
12821 Oak Hill Avenue
Hagerstown, MD 21742
Phone: 301-733-5971
Fax: 301-733-0872

Rockville

Shady Grove Sleep Disorders Center
14915 Broschart Road
Suite 260
Rockville, MD 20850
Phone: 301-251-5905
Fax: 301-251-6189

Massachusetts

Boston

Sleep Disorders Center
Beth Israel Deaconess Medical Center
330 Brookline Avenue, KS430
Boston, MA 02215
Phone: 617-667-3237
Fax: 617-975-5506
E-mail:
jmatheso@caregroup.harvard.edu

Burlington

Sleep Disorders Center
Lahey Clinic
41 Mall Road
Burlington, MA 01805
Phone: 781-744-8249
Fax: 781-744-5609
E-mail: **Ann.T.Wilkinson@Lahey.org**

Newton Center

Neurocare Inc./The Center for Sleep
Diagnostics
100 Wells Avenue
Suite 101
Newton Center, MA 02459
Phone: 617-796-7766
Fax: 617-796-9099
E-mail:
BQUINN@NEUROCAREINC.COM

Newton Center

Sleep HealthCenter
Affiliated with Brigham & Women's
Hospital
1400 Centre Street
Suite 109
Newton Center, MA 02459

Phone: 617-527-2227
Fax: 617-527-2098
E-mail:
**DAVID_WHITE@SLEEPHEALTH.
COM**
Web Site:
www.SLEEPHEALTH.COM

Salem

North Shore Sleep Center
North Shore Medical Center
81 Highland Avenue
Salem, MA 01970
Phone: 978-741-1215
Fax: 978-740-4901
E-mail: **sleeplab@nsmc.partners.org**

Worcester

Sleep Disorders Institute of Central
New England
St. Vincent Hospital at Worcester
Medical Center
20 Worcester Center Boulevard
Worcester, MA 01608
Phone: 508-363-6066 (Office) or
508-363-9485 (Lab)
Fax: 508-363-6373
E-mail:
Jayant.Phadke@tenethealth.com

Michigan

Ann Arbor

Michael S. Aldrich Sleep Disorders
Center
University of Michigan Hospitals
1500 East Medical Center Drive
UH8D 8702, Box 0117
Ann Arbor, MI 48109-0117
Phone: 734-936-9068

Fax: 734-936-5377
E-mail: **blivings@umich.edu**

Ann Arbor

Sleep Disorders Center
St. Joseph Mercy Hospital
PO Box 995
Ann Arbor, MI 48106
Phone: 734-712-4651
Fax: 734-712-2967

Bay City

sleep disorders center
bay medical center
1900 columbus avenue
bay city, mi 48708
phone: 517-894-3332
fax: 517-891-8164
e-mail: **marykay.taylor@bhsnet.org**
web site: **www.baymed.org**

Detroit

Sleep Disorders Center
Sinai-Grace Hospital
6071 West Outer Drive
Detroit, MI 48235
Phone: 313-966-3088
Fax: 313-966-1250
E-mail: **Rdobert@dmc.org**
Web Site: **www.sinaigrace.org/
sinaigrace/tour/sleepdisorder/**

Detroit

St. John Hospital Sleep Disorders
Center
St. John Hospital and Medical Center
22101 Moross Road
Detroit, MI 48236-2172
Phone: 313-343-7336

Fax: 313-343-3077
E-mail: **joann.maxim@stjohn.org**

Detroit

Sleep Disorders & Research Center
Henry Ford Health System
CFP3
2799 West Grand Boulevard
Detroit, MI 48202
Phone: 313-916-5174
Fax: 313-916-5150
E-mail: **dhudgel1@HFHS.ORG**

Detroit

Sleep/Wake Disorders Laboratory
(127B)
VA Medical Center
4646 John R. Street
Detroit, MI 48201-1916
Phone: 313-576-3663
Fax: 313-576-1377
E-mail:
SHELDON.KAPEN@MED.VA.GOV

Detroit

Sleep Disorders Center at Hutzel
Hospital
Hutzel Hospital
4707 St. Antoine, 1 Center
Detroit, MI 48201
Phone: 313-745-9009
Fax: 313-745-8725
E-mail: **jrowley@intmed.wayne.edu**

Flint

McLaren Sleep Diagnostic Center
McLaren Regional Medical Center
401 South Ballenger
Flint, MI 48532

Phone: 810-342-4980
Fax: 810-342-3655
E-mail: **kentm@mclaren.org**
Web Site: **www.mclaren.org**

Grand Rapids

Sleep Disorders Center at Spectrum
Health
4100 Lake Drive SE
Suite 100
Grand Rapids, MI 49546
Phone: 616-391-3759 or 888-
SLEEPLAB
Fax: 616-391-7879
E-mail: **ron.vandrunen@spectrum-
health.org**
Web Site: **www.spectrum-health.org/
centers/mss/sleep/default.asp**

Hastings

Sleep Disorders Center at
Pennock Hospital
1009 West Green Street
Hastings, MI 49058
Phone: 888-SLEEPLAB

Holland

Sleep Disorders Center at
Holland Community Hospital
602 Michigan Avenue
Holland, MI 49423
Phone: 888-SLEEPLAB

Iron Mountain

U.P. Sleep Disorders Center
Dickinson County Healthcare System
1711 South Stephenson Avenue
Iron Mountain, MI 49801

Phone: 906-776-5912
E-mail: **jcourney@dchs.org**

Jackson

Foote Hospital Sleep Disorders Center
W. A. Foote Memorial Hospital
205 North East Avenue
Jackson, MI 49201
Phone: 517-788-4750
Fax: 517-789-5968
E-mail: **pam.sayre@wafoote.org**

Kalamazoo

Sleep Disorders Center
Borgess Medical Center
1521 Gull Road
Kalamazoo, MI 49048
Phone: 616-226-7081
Fax: 616-226-6909
E-mail: **SheriDillon@Borgess.com**

Lansing

Ingham Regional Medical Center of
Sleep and Alertness
2727 South Pennsylvania Avenue
Lansing, MI 48910
Phone: 517-377-3525
Fax: 517-377-8530

Lansing

Sparrow Sleep Center
Sparrow Hospital
1200 East Michigan Avenue, Suite 455
PO Box 30480
Lansing, MI 48909-7980
Phone: 517-364-5370
Fax: 517-364-5373

Petoskey

1080 Hager Drive
NMH Sleep Center
Petoskey, MI 49770
Phone: 231-487-5337
Fax: 231-439-0059
E-mail: **ssmorch@northernhealth.org**

Southfield

Consultants in Sleep & Pulmonary
Medicine
28200 Franklin Road
Southfield, MI 48034
Phone: 248-350-2722
Fax: 248-350-0154

Traverse City

Munson Sleep Disorders Center
Munson Medical Center
1105 Sixth Street
MPB Suite 307
Traverse City, MI 49684-2386
Phone: 800-358-9641 or 231-935-
6600
Fax: 231-935-9300
E-mail: **MRINAL@MHC.NET**

Troy

Sleep Disorders Institute
44199 Dequindre
Suite 311
Troy, MI 48085
Phone: 248-879-0707
Fax: 248-879-2704
Web Site: **www.sleep-attention.com**

Warren

B.G. Tricounty Neurology & Sleep
Clinic
28111 Hoover
Suite 9A
Warren, MI 48093
Phone: 586-573-3750 or 888-922-
2233
Fax: 586-573-3756
E-mail:
BGTRICOUNTY@AOL.COM
Web Site: **SLEEPQUIET.COM**

Minnesota

Duluth

Duluth Regional Sleep Disorders
Center
St. Mary's Duluth Clinic Health System
407 East Third Street
Duluth, MN 55805
Phone: 218-786-4692
Fax: 218-786-4083
E-mail: **MCARLSON@SMDC.ORG**

Edina

Fairview Sleep Center
Fairview Southdale Hospital
6401 France Avenue South
Edina, MN 55435
Phone: 952-924-5053
Fax: 952-924-5994
E-mail:
RHOTTMA1@FAIRVIEW.ORG

Golden Valley

Minnesota Sleep Institute, Golden
Valley
Kindred Hospital

4101 Golden Valley Road
Golden Valley, MN 55443
Phone: 763-588-8796
Fax: 763-588-9081

Minneapolis

Minnesota Regional Sleep Disorders
Center, #868B
Hennepin County Medical Center
701 Park Avenue South
Minneapolis, MN 55415
Phone: 612-347-6288
Fax: 612-904-4207
E-mail:
MAHOW002@TC.UMN.EDU

Minneapolis

Sleep Disorders Center
Abbott Northwestern Hospital
800 East 28th Street at Chicago Avenue
Minneapolis, MN 55407
Phone: 612-863-4516
Fax: 612-863-2837
 Web Site:
www.abbottnorthwestern.com

Rochester

Mayo Sleep Disorders Center
Mayo Clinic
200 First Street SW
Rochester, MN 55905
Phone: 507-266-7456
Fax: 507-266-7772
E-mail: **sdcappointments@mayo.edu**

St. Paul

Metropolitan Sleep Disorders Center
LLP
255 North Smith Avenue

Suite 203
St. Paul, MN 55102
Phone: 651-298-0350
Fax: 651-298-0328

Mississippi

Columbus

Sleep Lab*
Baptist Memorial Hospital
2520 5th St. North
Columbus, MS 39701
Phone: 662-244-1176
Fax: 662-244-1293

Greenville

Sleep Disorders Laboratory*
The King's Daughters Hospital
300 South Washington Avenue
Greenville, MS 38701
Phone: 662-378-1118
Fax: 662-378-1134
E-mail: **tkdh-fbowman@hotmail.com**
Web Site: **www.tkdh.com**

Gulfport

Sleep Institute of the Gulf Coast
1110 Broad Avenue
Suite 600
Gulfport, MS 39501
Phone: 228-868-7593
Fax: 228-868-9930
Web Site: **snoozing.com**

Hattiesburg

Sleep Disorders Center
Forrest General Hospital
6051 Highway 49
PO Box 16389

Hattiesburg, MS 39404-6389
Phone: 601-288-1994 or 800-280-8520
Fax: 601-288-1999
E-mail: **sleeplab@forrestgeneral.com**
Web Site: **www.forrestgeneral.com**

Jackson

Sleep Disorder Center of Mississippi
Mississippi Baptist Medical Center
1225 North State Street
Jackson, MS 39202
Phone: 601-968-1157
Fax: 601-973-1653
E-mail: **gblatt@mbmc.org**
Web Site: **MBHS.org**

Jackson

Sleep Disorders Center and Division of Sleep Medicine
University of Mississippi Medical Center
2500 North State Street
Jackson, MS 39216-4505
Phone: 601-984-4820
Fax: 601-984-4828
E-mail:
hroffwarg@psychiatry.umsmed.edu
Web Site: **www2.umsmed.edu/dept/psych/SLEEP%20MEDICINE.htm**

Laurel

South Central Regional Medical Center
1220 Jefferson Street
Laurel, MS 39440
Phone: 601-426-4530
E-mail: **sleep@scrmc.com**

Meridian

Sleep Disorders Center
Jeff Anderson Regional Medical Center
2124 14th Street
Meridian, MS 39301
Phone: 601-553-6491
Fax: 601-553-6910
E-mail: **sleep-ms@netdoor.com**

Moss Point

Janice L. Miles, D.O.
Pulmonary & Sleep Medicine Sleep Lab*
3501 Main Street
Moss Point, MS 39563
Phone: 228-474-6111
Fax: 228-474-6113

Ocean Springs

Gulf Shore Sleep Disorders Center, LLC
22A Doctors Drive
Ocean Springs, MS 39564
Phone: 228-872-1951
Fax: 228-875-9998

Oxford

Sleep Disorder Center
Baptist Memorial Hospital—North Mississippi
2301 South Lamar
Oxford, MS 38655
Phone: 662-232-8146
Fax: 662-513-1694
E-mail: **kevin.buie@bmhcc.org**

Tupelo

Sleep Disorders Center
North Mississippi Medical Center
830 South Gloster Street
Tupelo, MS 38801
Phone: 662-377-3258
Fax: 662-377-2212
E-mail: **sleep@nmhs.net**
Web Site: **www.nmhs.net/
sleep_disorders/**

Missouri

Chesterfield

Sleep Medicine and Research Center
St. Luke's Hospital
232 South Woods Mill Road
Chesterfield, MO 63017
Phone: 314-205-6030
Fax: 314-205-6025
E-mail: **walsjk@stlo.smhs.com**

Columbia

University of Missouri Sleep Disorders
Center
M-178 Neurology
University Hospital and Clinics
One Hospital Drive
Columbia, MO 65212
Phone: 573-884-SLEEP or 800-ADD-
SLEEP
Fax: 573-884-4785
E-mail: **sahotap@health.missouri.edu**

Joplin

St. John's Sleep Disorders Center
St. John's Regional Medical Center
2727 McClelland Boulevard
Joplin, MO 64804

Phone: 417-625-2808
Fax: 417-659-6806
E-mail: **ameoli@stj.com**

Kansas City

Sleep Disorders Center
St. Luke's Hospital
4400 Wornall Road
Kansas City, MO 64111
Phone: 816-932-3207
Fax: 816-932-3383
E-mail: **ECOOK@SAINT-
LUKES.ORG**

Kansas City

Sleep Disorders Center
Research Medical Center
2316 East Meyer Boulevard
Kansas City, MO 64132-1199
Phone: 816-276-4334
Fax: 816-276-3488
E-mail: **jdmagee@healthmidwest.org**
Web Site: **www.healthmidwest.org**

Springfield

St. John's Sleep Disorders Center
St. John's Regional Health Center
1235 East Cherokee
Springfield, MO 65804
Phone: 417-885-5464
Fax: 417-885-5465

Springfield

Cox Regional Sleep Disorders Center
3800 South National Avenue
Suite LL 150
Springfield, MO 65807
Phone: 417-269-5575
Fax: 417-269-5578

E-mail: **Dave.Wortley@coxhealth.com**
Web Site: **www.COXHEALTH.COM**

St. Charles

St. Joseph Health Center Sleep
Disorders Laboratory*
St. Joseph Health Center
300 First Capitol Drive
St. Charles, MO 63301
Phone: 636-947-5165
Fax: 636-947-5164
E-mail: **thomas.siler.md@ssmhc.com**
Web Site: **www.ssmstjoseph.com**

St. Louis

Sleep Medicine Center
Washington University
212 North Kingshighway
Suite 237
St. Louis, MO 63108
Phone: 314-362-4342
Fax: 314-362-0296

Montana

Billings

The Sleep Center at St. Vincent
Hospital
St. Vincent Hospital and Health Center
1233 North 30th Street
Billings, MT 59101
Phone: 406-238-6815
Fax: 406-238-6262
E-mail: **wkohler@svh-mt.org**

Billings

Sleep Disorders Center
Deaconess Billings Clinic
2825 Eighth Avenue North

PO Box 37000
Billings, MT 59107
Phone: 406-238-2885
Fax: 406-238-2813
E-mail: **dsilbernagel@billingsclinic.org**
Web Site: **www.billingsclinic.org**

Great Falls

Rocky Mountain Sleep Disorders
Center, LLC
1917 Fourth Street South
Great Falls, MT 59405
Phone: 406-453-7570
Fax: 406-452-2566
E-mail: **rockymtnsleep@sofast.net**

Missoula

St. Patrick Hospital Sleep Center
St. Patrick Hospital
500 West Broadway
Missoula, MT 59802
Phone: 406-329-5650
Fax: 406-329-5605
E-mail: **Kenter@saintpatrick.org**
Web Site: **www.saintpatrick.org**

Nebraska

Lincoln

BryanLGH Center for Sleep Medicine
BryanLGH Medical Center West
2300 South 16th Street
Lincoln, NE 68502
Phone: 402-481-5338
Fax: 402-481-4831
E-mail: **leigh.heithoff@bryanlgh.org**

Lincoln

Adult and Pediatric Sleep Related
Breathing Disorders Laboratory*
BryanLGH Medical Center East
1600 South 48th Street
Lincoln, NE 68506
Phone: 402-481-3950
Fax: 402-481-8374
E-mail: **dbailey@bryanlgh.org**

Omaha

Sleep Disorders Center
Nebraska Health System
987546 Nebraska Medical Center
Omaha, NE 68198-7546
Phone: 402-552-2286
Fax: 402-552-2057

Omaha

Sleep Disorders Center
Methodist Hospital
2566 St. Mary's Avenue
Omaha, NE 68105
Phone: 402-354-6305 or 402-354-6309
Fax: 402-354-6334
E-mail: **tjbowman@pol.net**

Papillion

Sleep & Breathing Disorders Lab*
Alegent Health Midlands Medical
Center
11111 South 84th Street
Papillion, NE 68046
Phone: 402-593-3720
Fax: 402-593-3725
E-mail: **sseiberl@alegent.org**

Nevada

Carson City

Mountain Medical Sleep Disorders
Center
Mountain Medical Associates, Inc.
710 West Washington Street
Carson City, NV 89703-3826
Phone: 775-882-2106 or 775-882-4139
Fax: 775-882-0838
E-mail: **DZIMMER889@AOL.COM**

Henderson

The Sleep Clinic of Nevada at St. Rose
Dominican Hospital
102 East Lake Mead Drive
Henderson, NV 89105
Phone: 702-893-0020
Fax: 702-893-0025

Las Vegas

Regional Center for Sleep Disorders
Sunrise Hospital and Medical Center
3131 LaCanada, Suite 107
Las Vegas, NV 89109
Phone: 702-731-8365
Fax: 702-731-8978

Las Vegas

Regional Center for Sleep
Disorders—West
Sunrise Hospital and Medical Center
3150 North Tenaya Way, Suite 115
Las Vegas, NV 89218
Phone: 702-255-5040
Fax: 702-255-5196

Las Vegas

The Sleep Clinic of Nevada
1012 East Sahara Avenue
Las Vegas, NV 89104
Phone: 702-893-0020
Fax: 702-893-0025
E-mail: **thesleepclinician@aol.com**

Reno

Washoe Sleep Disorders Center and
Sleep Laboratory
Sleep Management, Inc.,
EYE-COM, Inc.
Washoe Professional Building and
Washoe Medical Center
75 Pringle Way, Suite 701
Reno, NV 89502
Phone: 775-329-4060
Fax: 775-329-2715
E-mail: **EYECOMM@AOL.COM**

Reno

Pulmonary Medicine Associates Sleep
Center
601 South Arlington Avenue
Reno, NV 89509
Phone: 775-329-1727
Fax: 775-329-4016

New Hampshire

Lebanon

Sleep Disorders Center
Dartmouth-Hitchcock Medical Center
One Medical Center Drive
Lebanon, NH 03756
Phone: 603-650-7534
Fax: 603-650-7820

E-mail:
sleep.disorders.center@dartmouth.edu

Manchester

Center for Sleep Evaluation
Elliot Hospital
One Elliot Way
Manchester, NH 03103
Phone: 603-663-6680
Fax: 603-663-6699

New Jersey

Dover

Center for Sleep Medicine
Saint Clare's Hospital
400 West Blackwell Street
Dover, NJ 07801
Phone: 973-989-3477
Fax: 973-989-3478
E-mail: **sfitzgerald@saintclares.org**
Web Site: **www.saintclares.org** or
mjatkins.salu.net

Edison

Center for Sleep Disorders Treatment,
Research & Education
New Jersey Neuroscience Institute at
JFK Medical Center
65 James Street
Edison, NJ 08818
Phone: 732-321-7935
Fax: 732-205-1477
E-mail:
KRAHMAN@SOLARISHS.ORG

Hackensack

Institute for Sleep/Wake Disorders
Hackensack University Medical Center

30 Prospect Avenue
Hackensack, NJ 07601
Phone: 201-996-3732
Fax: 201-498-1163

Morristown

Sleep Disorder Center
Morristown Memorial Hospital
95 Mount Kemble Avenue
Morristown, NJ 07962
Phone: 973-971-4567
Fax: 973-290-7620
Web Site: **www.atlantichealth.org**

Mount Holly

SleepCare
Virtua Health
175 Madison Avenue
Mount Holly, NJ 08060
Phone: 800-753-3779
Fax: 856-234-5010
E-mail:
**JMILADIN@SLEEPCARECENTER.
COM**
Web Site: **sleepcarecenter.com**

Mount Laurel

SleepCare Centers, Inc.
130 Gaither Drive, Suite 124
Mount Laurel, NJ 08054
Phone: 800-753-3779
Fax: 856-234-5010
E-mail:
**JMILADIN@SLEEPCARECENTER.
COM**
Web Site: **sleepcarecenter.com**

New Brunswick

Comprehensive Sleep Disorders Center
Robert Wood Johnson University
Hospital/
UMDNJ—Robert Wood Johnson
Medical School
One Robert Wood Johnson Place, PO
Box 2601
New Brunswick, NJ 08903-2601
Phone: 732-937-8683
Fax: 732-418-8448

Newark

Sleep Disorders Center
Newark Beth Israel Medical Center
201 Lyons Avenue
Newark, NJ 07112
Phone: 973-926-6668
Fax: 973-923-6672
E-mail: **MKARETZK@sbhcs.com**
Web Site: **www.njsleephelp.com**

Scotch Plains

Sleep Disorders Center of New Jersey
2253 South Avenue, Suite 7
Scotch Plains, NJ 07076
Phone: 908-789-4244
Fax: 908-789-2716
E-mail: **mail@sleepNJ.com**
Web Site: **www.SleepNJ.com**

Trenton

Snoring and Sleep Apnea Center of
Mercer County
Capital Health System
750 Brunswick Avenue
Trenton, NJ 08638
Phone: 609-278-6990
Fax: 609-278-6982

E-mail: **Rbrooks@chsnj.org**
Web Site: **www.capitalhealth.org**

Trenton

Sleep Disorder Program
St. Francis Medical Center
601 Hamilton Avenue
Trenton, NJ 08629
Phone: 609-599-6206
Fax: 609-599-6275
E-mail: **TGALLOWAY@CHE-EAST.ORG**
Web Site: **www.stfrancismedical.org**

Trenton

Mercer Sleep Disorders Center
Capital Health System
446 Bellevue Avenue
Trenton, NJ 08607
Phone: 609-394-4167
Fax: 609-394-4352
E-mail: **Rbrooks@chsnj.org**

New Mexico

Albuquerque

New Mexico Center for Sleep Medicine
Lovelace Health Systems
4700 Jefferson NE, Suite 800
Albuquerque, NM 87109
Phone: 505-872-6000 or Toll Free:
887-805-REST
Fax: 505-872-6003
E-mail:
NLPOLN@LOVELACE.COM
Web Site: **www.LOVELACE.COM**

Albuquerque

University Hospital Sleep Disorders
Center
4775 Indian School Road NE,
Suite 303
Albuquerque, NM 87110
Phone: 505-272-6110
Fax: 505-272-6112
E-mail: **mrdavidson@salud.unm.edu**

New York

Albany

Capital Region Sleep/Wake Disorders
Center
St. Peter's Hospital
Pine West Plaza #1
Washington Avenue Extension
Albany, NY 12205
Phone: 518-464-9999
Fax: 518-464-9650
E-mail:
**SLEEP@STPETERSHEALTHCARE.
ORG**
Web Site:
**www.STPETERSHEALTHCARE.
ORG**

Binghamton

Sleep Disorders Center
United Health Services
33 Mitchell Avenue, Suite 115
Binghamton, NY 13903
Phone: 607-762-2048
Fax: 607-762-2051
E-mail:
SLEEP_CENTER@UHS.ORG

Bronx

Sleep Disorders Center
Montefiore Medical Center
111 East 210th Street

Bronx, NY 10467
Phone: 718-920-4841
Fax: 718-798-4352
E-mail: **Thorpy@aecom.yu.edu**
Web Site: **www.cloud9.net/~thorpy/
mmc/**

Brooklyn

North Shore Long Island Jewish Sleep
Center at Brooklyn
387 Clinton Street
Brooklyn, NY 11231
Phone: 718-470-7958
Fax: 718-470-1035
E-mail: **greenber@lij.edu**

Brooklyn

Sleep Disorders Center
New York Methodist Hospital
506 Sixth Street
Brooklyn, NY 11215
Phone: 718-780-3017
Fax: 718-780-6711

Buffalo

Sleep Disorder Center of Western
New York
Kaleida Health
3 Gates Circle
Buffalo, NY 14222
Phone: 716-88-SLEEP (887-5337)
Fax: 716-887-5332
E-mail: **drifkin@kaleidahealth.org**

Cooperstown

Bassett Healthcare Sleep Disorders
Center
Bassett Healthcare
One Atwell Road

Cooperstown, NY 13326
Phone: 607-547-6979
Fax: 607-547-6906
E-mail: **bob.reese@bassett.org**
Web Site: **www.bassetthealthcare.org**

Elmira

St. Joseph's Hospital Sleep Disorders
Center
St. Joseph's Hospital
555 East Market Street
Elmira, NY 14902
Phone: 607-737-7008
Fax: 607-271-3410
E-mail: **webmaster@stjosephs.org**
Web Site: **www.stjosephs.org**

Forest Hills

Parkway Hospital Sleep Disorders
Center
The Parkway Hospital
70-35 113th Street
Forest Hills, NY 11375
Phone: 718-990-4590
Fax: 718-268-6110
E-mail: **info@phsdc.com**
Web Site: **www.phsdc.com**

Great Neck

North Shore Long Island Jewish Sleep
Center
155 Community Drive
Great Neck, NY 11021
Phone: 516-465-8271 or 877-
SLEEPMD
Fax: 516-465-8299
E-mail: **GREENBER@LIJ.EDU**

Hornell

Sleep Disorders Laboratory*
St. James Mercy Health
411 Canisteo Street
Hornell, NY 14843
Phone: 607-324-8781
Fax: 607-324-8785

Mineola

Sleep Disorders Center
Winthrop-University Hospital
222 Station Plaza North
Mineola, NY 11501
Phone: 516-663-3907
Fax: 516-663-4788
E-mail: mweinstein@winthrop.org

New York

The Sleep Disorders Center
New York-Presbyterian Hospital
Columbia-Presbyterian Medical Center
161 Fort Washington Avenue
New York, NY 10032
Phone: 212-305-1860
Fax: 212-305-5496
E-mail: NBK1@COLUMBIA.EDU
Web Site: www.sleepnyp.com

New York

Clinlabs, Inc.
Sleep Disorders Institute
1090 Amsterdam Avenue
New York, NY 10025
Phone: 212-523-1700 or 888-
SLEEPNY
Fax: 212-523-1704
E-mail: gzammit@clinilabs.com
Web Site: www.clinilabs.com

Rochester

Sleep Disorders Center of Rochester
2110 Clinton Avenue South
Rochester, NY 14618
Phone: 585-442-4141
Fax: 585-442-6259
Web Site: www.unityhealth.org/
unitynow/sleepdisorders.html

Staten Island

Sleep Apnea Center*
Staten Island University Hospital
375 Seguine Avenue
Staten Island, NY 10309
Phone: 800-333-6533 or 718-226-
2331
Fax: 718-226-2735
E-mail: sgrenard@siuh.edu
Web Site: www.siuh.edu/sleeplab

Stony Brook

Sleep Disorders Center
State University of New York at
Stony Brook
University Hospital
MR 120A
Stony Brook, NY 11794-7139
Phone: 631-444-2916
Fax: 631-444-7851
E-mail: mmaczaj@mail-
psychiatry.sunysb.edu
Web Site:
SleepDisordersCenter.UHMC.SUNYS
B.edu

Syracuse

The Sleep Laboratory
St. Joseph's Hospital Health Center
945 East Genesee Street, Suite 300

Syracuse, NY 13210
Phone: 315-475-3379
Fax: 315-475-5077
Web Site: **www.SJHSYR.ORG**

Syracuse

The Sleep Center
Community General Hospital
Broad Road
Syracuse, NY 13215
Phone: 315-492-5877
Fax: 315-492-5521
Web Site: **www.cgh.org**

Utica

The Mohawk Valley Sleep Disorders
Center at
St. Elizabeth Medical Center
2209 Genesee Street
Utica, NY 13501
Phone: 315-734-3484
Fax: 315-734-3494
E-mail: **mvsdc@stemc.org**

Watertown

Sleep Disorders Center of Northern
New York
Samaritan Medical Center
830 Washington Street
Watertown, NY 13601
Phone: 315-786-4930
Fax: 315-786-4933
E-mail: **caloan@shsny.com**
Web Site: **www.samaritanhealth.com**

White Plains

The Sleep Disorders Center-
White Plains
New York-Presbyterian Hospital

Columbia-Presbyterian Medical Center
185 Maple Avenue
White Plains, NY 10601
Phone: 914-948-0400
Fax: 212-305-5496
E-mail: **NBK1@COLUMBIA.EDU**
Web Site: **www.sleepnyp.com**

White Plains

Sleep-Wake Disorders Center
The New York Presbyterian
Hospital—Westchester Division
21 Bloomingdale Road
White Plains, NY 10605
Phone: 914-997-5751
Fax: 914-682-6911
E-mail: **mmoline@med.cornell.edu**

North Carolina

Asheville

Mission/St. Joseph's Sleep Center
445 Biltmore Avenue, Suite 404
Asheville, NC 28801
Phone: 828-213-4670
Fax: 828-213-4672

Charlotte

Carolinas Sleep Services
Mercy Hospital South
16028 Park Road
Charlotte, NC 28210
Phone: 704-543-2213
Fax: 704-341-6848
E-mail: **mstolzenbach@carolinas.org**

Charlotte

Novant Sleep Services
Presbyterian Healthcare

1900 Randolph Road, Suite 300
Charlotte, NC 28207
Phone: 704-384-6225
Fax: 704-384-6264
E-mail: **remiller@novanthealth.org**
Web Site: **www.presbyterian.org** &
www. novantsleep.com

Charlotte

Carolinas Sleep Services
University Hospital
PO Box 560727
8800 North Tyron Street
Charlotte, NC 28256
Phone: 704-548-5855 or 877-
2SLEEPEZ
Fax: 704-548-5891
E-mail: **mstolzenbach@carolinas.org**
Web Site: **www.carolinas.org**

Greensboro

Sleep Disorders Center
Moses Cone Health System
501 North Elam Avenue
Greensboro, NC 27403
Phone: 336-832-0410
Fax: 336-832-0411

Greenville

Sleep Disorders Center
Pitt County Memorial Hospital
University Health Systems of Eastern
North Carolina
#4 Doctor's Park Medical Drive
Greenville, NC 27834
Phone: 252-744-7502
Fax: 252-744-7505
E-mail: **gedwards@pcmh.com**
Web Site: **www.uhseast.com**

Hendersonville

Sleep Center of Pardee
Margaret R. Pardee Hospital
715 Fleming Street
Hendersonville, NC 28791
Phone: 828-696-1085
Fax: 828-696-1081
E-mail: **terry.weldon@pardee-med.org**
Web Site: **www.pardee-med.org**

Salisbury

Sleep Medicine Center of Salisbury
911 West Henderson Street
Suite L30
Salisbury, NC 28144
Phone: 704-637-1533
Fax: 704-637-0470
E-mail: **hill@2sleepy.com**

Statesville

Summit Sleep Center—Statesville
760 Hartness Road
Statesville, NC 28677
Phone: 704-878-0358
Fax: 704-878-0703
E-mail:
BALDWINSMITHIII@Prodigy.net

Winston-Salem

Summit Sleep Disorders Center
160 Charlois Boulevard
Winston-Salem, NC 27103
Phone: 336-765-5834
Fax: 336-765-4889
E-mail:
BALDWINSMITHIII@prodigy.net

Winston-Salem

Sleep Disorders Center
North Carolina Baptist Hospital
Wake Forest University School of
Medicine
Medical Center Boulevard
Winston-Salem, NC 27157
Phone: 336-716-5288
Fax: 336-716-9742
E-mail: **vmcall@wfubmc.edu**
Web Site: **www.wfubmc.edu**

North Dakota

Fargo

MeritCare Sleep Disorders Center
MeritCare Health Center
720 N 4th Street
Fargo, ND 58122
Phone: 701-234-5673
Fax: 701-234-7195

Ohio

Akron

Sleep Disorders Center
Akron General Medical Center
400 Wabash Avenue
Akron, OH 44307
Phone: 330-344-6751
Fax: 330-344-6186
E-mail: **rleon@agmc.org**

Akron

Sleep Disorders Center
Akron General Medical Center
4073 Medina Road
Akron, OH 44333

Phone: 330-344-6751
Fax: 330-344-6186

Canton

Mercy Sleep Center
Mercy Medical Center
1320 Mercy Drive NW
Canton, OH 44708
Phone: 330-489-1456
Fax: 330-489-6039
E-mail:
karen.lehmiller@cahealthcare.com

Cincinnati

The Tri-State Sleep Disorders Center
1275 East Kemper Road
Cincinnati, OH 45246
Phone: 513-671-3101
Fax: 513-671-4159
E-mail: **SleepSatl@aol.com**

Cincinnati

Cincinnati Regional Sleep Centers
2123 Auburn Avenue
Suite 334
Cincinnati, OH 45219
Phone: 513-721-4680
Fax: 513-721-1036
E-mail: **CRSC@fuse.net**
Web Site:
www.cincinnatisleepcenter.com

Cincinnati

TriHealth Sleep and Alertness Center
Good Samaritan Hospital
375 Dixmyth Avenue—7H
Cincinnati, OH 45220-2489
Phone: 513-872-4000
Fax: 513-872-7873

E-mail: virgil_wooten@trihealth.com
Web Site: www.trihealth.org

Cincinnati

Cincinnati Regional Sleep
Centers—West
5049 Crookshank Road
Suite G-3
Cincinnati, OH 45238
Phone: 513-347-0220
Fax: 513-347-5173
E-mail: CRSC@fuse.net
Web Site: cincinnatisleepcenter.com

Cleveland

Sleep Disorders Center
The Cleveland Clinic Foundation
9500 Euclid Avenue
Desk S-51
Cleveland, OH 44195
Phone: 216-444-2165
Fax: 216-445-6205
E-mail: foldvan@ccf.org
Web Site: www.clevelandclinic.org/
neurology

Cleveland

West Region Sleep Center
15805 Puritas Avenue
Cleveland, OH 44135
Phone: 216-267-5933
Fax: 216-267-5133
E-mail:
SLEEPLAB@OHIOCHEST.COM

Cleveland

University Hospitals Sleep Center
University Hospitals of Cleveland
Department of Neurology

11100 Euclid Avenue
Cleveland, OH 44106
Phone: 216-844-1301
Fax: 216-844-8753

Cleveland

Sleep Disorders Program
MetroHealth Medical Center
2500 MetroHealth Drive
Cleveland, OH 44109
Phone: 216-778-5984
Fax: 216-778-8215
E-mail: dauckley@metrohealth.org

Columbus

Eastside Sleep Diagnostic Center
81 Outerbelt Street
Columbus, OH 43213
Phone: 614-751-2141
Fax: 614-866-9131
E-mail: jheffern@ohiohealth.com
Web Site: www.ohiohealth.com

Columbus

Worthington Sleep Wake Center
7811 Flint Road
Suite D
Columbus, OH 43235
Phone: 614-848-4198
Fax: 614-848-3717
E-mail: sholt@gradyhospital.com

Columbus

Riverside Methodist Hospital Sleep
Center
Riverside Methodist Hospital
3535 Olentangy River Road
Columbus, OH 43214
Phone: 614-566-5270

Fax: 614-566-6877
E-mail: **Rickmam@ohiohealth.com**

Columbus

Regional Sleep Disorder Center
Columbus Community Health
1430 South High Street
Columbus, OH 43207
Phone: 614-443-7800
Fax: 614-443-6960
E-mail: **flamenco@netexp.net**
Web Site: **www.thesleepsite.com**

Dayton

Sleep Disorders Center
Kettering Medical Center
3535 Southern Boulevard
Dayton, OH 45429-1295
Phone: 937-395-8805
Fax: 937-395-8821
E-mail:
Donna.Arand@kmcnetwork.org

Dayton

The Center for Sleep & Wake
Disorders
Miami Valley Hospital
One Wyoming Street
Suite G-200
Dayton, OH 45409
Phone: 937-208-2515
Fax: 937-208-5685
E-mail: **KMHUBAN@MVH.ORG**

Dayton

Samaritan North Sleep Laboratory*
9000 North Main Street
Suite 225
Dayton, OH 45415

Phone: 937-567-6180
Fax: 937-567-6187
E-mail: **Jgray@SHP_Dayton.org**

Delaware

Sleep Disorders Center
Grady Memorial Hospital
561 West Central Avenue
Delaware, OH 43015
Phone: 740-368-5330
Fax: 740-368-5331
E-mail: **sholt@gradyhospital.com**

Dublin

Ohio Sleep Medicine Institute
4975 Bradenton Avenue
Dublin, OH 43017
Phone: 614-766-0773
Fax: 614-766-2599
E-mail: **sleepohio@aol.com**
Web Site: **www.sleepohio.com**

Gahanna

Central Ohio Sleep Medicine
Mount Carmel Hospital & Central
Ohio Pulmonary Disease
4625 Morse Road
Suite 200
Gahanna, OH 43230
Phone: 614-475-6700
Fax: 614-475-6800
E-mail: **JACounts@aol.com**

Gallipolis

Sleep Disorders Laboratory*
Holzer Clinic
90 Jackson Pike
Gallipolis, OH 45631
Phone: 740-446-5525

Fax: 740-446-5565
E-mail: **Hlinder@holzerclinic.com**

Garfield Heights

Marymount Hospital Sleep Disorders
Center
Marymount Hospital
12300 McCracken Road
Garfield Heights, OH 44125
Phone: 216-587-8151
Fax: 216-587-8857
E-mail: **gforeman@marymount.org**

Lima

St. Rita's Sleep Disorders Lab*
St. Rita's Medical Center
730 West Market Street
Lima, OH 45801
Phone: 419-226-9397
Fax: 419-226-9535
E-mail: **mreed@health-partners.org**

Mason

Sleepcare Diagnostics
4700 Duke Drive, Suite 180
Mason, OH 45040
Phone: 513-459-7750
Fax: 513-459-8030
E-mail: **jim@snorenomore.com**
Web Site: **www.snorenomore.com**

Maumee

Sleep Disorders Center
St. Luke's Hospital
5901 Monclova Road
Maumee, OH 43537
Phone: 419-897-8490
Fax: 419-897-8491
Web Site: **www.stlukeshospital.com**

Mayfield Heights

Sleep Disorders Center
Hillcrest Hospital
6780 Mayfield Road
Mayfield Heights, OH 44124
Phone: 440-646-8090
Fax: 440-460-2805
E-mail: **sleeplab@meridia.org**
Web Site: **www.sleeplab@meridia.org**

Medina

MGH Sleep Related Breathing
Disorders Lab*
Medina General Hospital
1000 East Washington Street
Medina, OH 44256
Phone: 330-725-1000 x2350
Fax: 330-721-4927
E-mail: **mmillsap@medinahospital.org**

Montrose

Ohio Sleep Disorders Center
150 Springside Drive
Montrose, OH 44333
Phone: 330-670-1290
Fax: 330-670-1292

Oregon

Sleep Disorders Center
St. Charles Mercy Hospital
2600 Navarre Avenue
Oregon, OH 43616
Phone: 419-696-7100
Fax: 419-696-7102
E-mail: **James_Kusina@mhsnr.org**
Web Site: **www.mercyweb.org**

Sylvania

Northwest Ohio Sleep Disorders Center
at Flower Hospital
5200 Harroun Road
Sylvania, OH 43560
Phone: 419-824-1624
Fax: 419-824-1638
E-mail: **pamlang@promedica.org**

Tiffin

Sleep Improvement Lab*
Mercy Hospital Tiffin
PO Box 727
Tiffin, OH 44883-0727
Phone: 419-448-7666
Fax: 419-448-7669
E-mail: **lynette_clifton@mhsnr.org**

Toledo

Northwest Ohio Sleep Disorders Center
The Toledo Hospital
Harris-McIntosh Tower, Second Floor
2142 North Cove Boulevard
Toledo, OH 43606
Phone: 419-291-5629
Fax: 419-479-6954

Toledo

Sleep Disorders Center
St. Vincent Medical Center
3829 Woodley, Suite 1
Toledo, OH 43606
Phone: 419-251-0570
Fax: 419-251-0574
E-mail: **mneeb@hotmail.com**

Uniontown

Ohio Sleep Disorders Centers—Green
1700 Boettler Road, Suite 250
Uniontown, OH 44685-7794
Phone: 330-498-5020
Fax: 330-498-5022

Zanesville

Sleep Disorders Center
Genesis Health Care System
Bethesda Hospital
2951 Maple Avenue
Zanesville, OH 43701
Phone: 740-454-4725
Fax: 740-450-6168
Web Site: www. genesishcs.org/

Oklahoma

Oklahoma City

Sleep Disorders Center of Oklahoma
Integris Health
4401 South Western Avenue
Oklahoma City, OK 73109
Phone: 405-636-7700
Fax: 405-636-7531
E-mail: **veitca@integris-health.com**
Web Site: **www.integris-health.com**

Oklahoma City

Sleep Disorders Center of Oklahoma
Integris Baptist Medical Center
3300 Northwest Expressway
Oklahoma City, OK 73112
Phone: 405-951-8333
Fax: 405-636-7531
E-mail: **veitca@integris-health.com**

Oregon

Bend

High Desert Sleep Disorders
Laboratory*
2042 Williamson Court
Bend, OR 97701
Phone: 541-383-6905
Fax: 541-383-6906
E-mail: **G.Calliso@smsc.org**

Eugene

Sleep Disorders & Neurology Clinic
4725 Village Plaza Coop
Suite 101
Eugene, OR 97401
Phone: 541-683-3325
Fax: 541-343-4117
E-mail: **SDNClinic@hotmail.com**

Eugene

Sleep Disorders Center
Sacred Heart Medical Center
1255 Hilyard Street
PO Box 10905
Eugene, OR 97440
Phone: 503-686-7224
Fax: 503-686-3765
E-mail: **CDunks@peacehealth.org**

Medford

Sleep Disorders Center
Rogue Valley Medical Center
2825 East Barnett Road
Medford, OR 97504
Phone: 541-608-4320
Fax: 541-608-5890
E-mail: **GZANOTTO@asante.org**

Portland

Pacific Sleep Program
1849 Northwest Kearney
Suite 202
Portland, OR 97209
Phone: 503-228-4414
Fax: 503-228-7293
E-mail: **Sleep@snoreweb.com**
Web Site: **www.snoreweb.com**

Portland

Sleep Disorders Center
Providence St. Vincent Medical Center
9205 Southwest Barnes Road
Portland, OR 97225
Phone: 503-216-2010
Fax: 503-216-2614
E-mail: **lmiskowicz@providence.org**

Portland

Sleep Disorders Center
Providence Portland Medical Center
4805 Northeast Glisan Street
Portland, OR 97213-1967
Phone: 503-215-3095
Fax: 503-215-2993
E-mail: **dhurst@providence.org**

Portland

Legacy Good Samaritan Sleep Disorders
Center
1015 Northwest 22nd Avenue
Suite 315
Portland, OR 97210
Phone: 503-413-7540
Fax: 503-413-6919

Salem

Salem Hospital Sleep Disorders Center
Salem Hospital
875 Oak Street SE
PO Box 14001
Salem, OR 97309-5014
Phone: 503-561-5170
Fax: 503-561-4709
E-mail: **SJBaug@SalemHospital.org**
Web Site: **www.salemhospital.org/
services/sleepdisorder.html**

The Dalles

MCMC Sleep Studies Lab
Mid-Columbia Medical Center
1700 East 19th Street
The Dalles, OR 97058
Phone: 541-296-7724
Fax: 547-296-7605
E-mail: **MichaelW@mcmc.net**

Pennsylvania

Allentown

Lehigh Valley Hospital Sleep Disorders
Center
Lehigh Valley Hospital
17th & Chew Streets
Allentown, PA 18103
Phone: 610-402-9777
Fax: 610-402-9770
E-mail: **Richard.Strobel@lvh.com**

Allentown

Sacred Heart Sleep Disorders Center
Sacred Heart Hospital
421 Chew Street
Allentown, PA 18102-3490
Phone: 610-776-5333

Fax: 610-776-5110
E-mail: **SHH_SLEEP@JUNO.COM**

Altoona

Institute for Sleep Medicine
Bon Secours—Holy Family Hospital
2500 Seventh Avenue
Altoona, PA 16630
Phone: 814-949-4466
Fax: 814-949-5893
E-mail: **jyounger@keyconn.net**
Web Site:
**www.bonsecoursholyfamily.org/
sleepnet.htm**

Bristol

Sleep Disorders Center
Temple Lower Bucks Hospital
501 Bath Road
Bristol, PA 19007
Phone: 215-785-9752
Fax: 215-785-9068

Carlisle

Carlisle Regional Medical Center Sleep
Center
Carlisle Hospital
Box 4100
246 Parker Street
Carlisle, PA 17013
Phone: 717-245-5838
Fax: 717-245-5836
E-mail:
**SLEEPLAB@CRMCPA.HMA_CORP
.COM**
Web Site: **www.carlisleRMC.com**

Danville

Geisinger Medical Center Sleep
Disorders Center
Geisinger Medical Center
100 North Academy Avenue
Danville, PA 17821
Phone: 570-271-6508
Fax: 570-271-7143
E-mail: **apmatragrano@geisinger.edu**

Doylestown

Penn Sleep Centers: Doylestown
800 West State Street
Doylestown, PA 18901
Phone: 215-662-7772
Fax: 215-349-8038
E-mail:
Samantha.Cartegena@uphs.upenn.edu

Lafayette Hill

Center for Sleep Medicine
443 Germantown Pike
Lafayette Hill, PA 19444
Phone: 610-828-4060
Fax: 610-238-5300

Lancaster

Sleep Disorders Center of Lancaster
Lancaster General Hospital
555 North Duke Street
Lancaster, PA 17604-3555
Phone: 717-290-5910
Fax: 717-290-4592
E-mail:
jmoconno@lancastergeneral.org
Web Site: **www.lancastergeneral.com**

Langhorne

Saint Mary Sleep/Wake Disorder
Center
Langhorne-Newtown Road
Langhorne, PA 19047
Phone: 215-741-6744
Fax: 215-741-6695

Meadowbrook

Holy Redeemer Sleep Disorders Lab*
Holy Redeemer Hospital and Medical
Center
1648 Huntingdon Pike
Meadowbrook, PA 19046
Phone: 215-938-3448
Fax: 215-938-3958
E-mail: **lt00@Holyredeemer.com**

Paoli

Sleep Medicine Services
Paoli Memorial Hospital
255 West Lancaster Avenue
Paoli, PA 19301
Phone: 610-645-3400
Fax: 610-645-2291
E-mail: **pressmanm@MLHS.org**

Philadelphia

Penn Sleep Centers
Hospital of the University of
Pennsylvania
3400 Spruce Street
11 Gates West
Philadelphia, PA 19104
Phone: 215-662-7772
Fax: 215-349-8038
E-mail:
Samantha.Cartagena@uphs.upenn.edu

Philadelphia

Northeast Sleep Disorders Center
Nazareth Hospital
2601 Holme Avenue
Philadelphia, PA 19152
Phone: 215-335-6190
Fax: 215-335-6182

Philadelphia

sleep disorders center
thomas jefferson university
1015 walnut street
suite 319
philadelphia, pa 19107
phone: 215-955-6175
fax: 215-955-9783
e-mail: **karl.doghramji@mail.tju.edu**
web site: **www.jeffersonhealth.org/tjuh/
centers/sleep/index.html**

Philadelphia

Penn Sleep Centers: Presbyterian
Medical Center
Scheie 405
51 North 39th Street
Philadelphia, PA 19104
Phone: 215-662-8863
Fax: 215-349-8038
E-mail: **bstaley@mail.med.upenn.edu**

Philadelphia

Pennsylvania Hospital Sleep Disorders
Center
Pennsylvania Hospital
Eighth and Spruce Streets
Philadelphia, PA 19107
Phone: 215-829-7079
Fax: 215-829-5630

Web Site: **www.uphs.edu/pahosp/hs-
files/neurology/sleep-dis.html**

Philadelphia

Temple University Health System Sleep
Disorders Center
at Temple University Hospital
3401 North Broad Street
7th Floor, Parkinson Pavilion
Philadelphia, PA 19140
Phone: 215-707-8163
Fax: 215-707-8167
E-mail:
DenaulGr@TUHS.Temple.edu

Philadelphia

University Services
5301 Tacony Street
Philadelphia, PA 19137
Phone: 215-743-4200
Fax: 215-743-7786
E-mail: **sleepinfo@uservices.com**
Web Site: **www.uservices.com**

Pittsburgh

Sleep Evaluation Center
Western Psychiatric Institute and Clinic
3811 O'Hara Street
Pittsburgh, PA 15213-2593
Phone: 412-624-2246
Fax: 412-624-2841

Pottstown

University Services
1133 High Street
Pottstown, PA 19464
Phone: 610-326-6737
Fax: 610-326-7551

E-mail: **MMISERO@CHESCO.COM**
Web Site: **www.uservices.com**

Ridley Park

Crozer Sleep Disorders Center at Taylor
Hospital
175 East Chester Pike
Ridley Park, PA 19078
Phone: 610-595-6272
Fax: 610-595-6273
E-mail: **staffordt@dvol.com**

Scranton

Sleep Disorders Center
Community Medical Center
1822 Mulberry Street
Scranton, PA 18510
Phone: 570-969-8931

Washington

Washington Hospital Sleep Center
The Washington Hospital
155 Wilson
Washington, PA 15301
Phone: 724-223-3287
Fax: 724-229-2400
E-mail:
fgladysz@washingtonhospital.org

Wilkes-Barre

Sleep Disorders Center
Mercy Hospital
25 Church Street
Wilkes-Barre, PA 18765
Phone: 570-826-3410
Fax: 570-820-6658

Wynnewood

Sleep Medicine Services
The Lankenau Hospital
100 Lancaster Avenue
Wynnewood, PA 19096
Phone: 610-645-3400
Fax: 610-642-2291
E-mail: **pressmanm@MLHS.org**

Wyomissing

Eastern Pennsylvania Comprehensive
Sleep Disorders Center
867 Berkshire Boulevard, Suite 100
Wyomissing, PA 19610
Phone: 610-378-5566
Fax: 610-378-5470
E-mail: **stanfordmd@mindspring.com**
Web Site:
www.easternpafeinberg.baweb.com

Rhode Island

Newport

Sleep Disorders Center of Lifespan
Hospitals-Newport Hospital
Newport Hospital
East Wing
11 Friendship Street
Newport, RI 02840
Phone: 401-444-4269
Fax: 401-444-8720

Providence

Sleep Disorders Center of Lifespan
Hospitals
Miriam Hospital
164 Summit Avenue
Providence, RI 02906

Phone: 401-444-4269
Fax: 401-444-8720

Providence

Sleep Disorders Center of Lifespan
Hospitals
Rhode Island Hospital
APC 301
593 Eddy Street
Providence, RI 02903
Phone: 401-444-4269
Fax: 401-444-8720
E-mail: **gkipp@lifespan.org**

South Carolina

Charleston

Roper Sleep/Wake Disorders Center
Roper Hospital
316 Calhoun Street
Charleston, SC 29401-1125
Phone: 843-724-2246
Fax: 843-724-2765
E-mail: **tim.fultz@carealliance.com**
Web Site: **www.carealliance.com/sleep/
index.html**

Columbia

Sleep Med of South Carolina
Baptist Medical Center
Taylor at Marion Streets
Columbia, SC 29220
Phone: 803-296-5847 or 800-368-
1971
Fax: 803-296-3080
Web Site: **www.sleepmed.md**

Easley

Southeast Regional Sleep Disorders
Center Easley
200 Fleetwood Drive
PO Box 2129
Easley, SC 29640
Phone: 864-855-7200
Fax: 864-627-9301

Greenville

Southeast Regional Sleep Disorders
Center
440A Roper Mountain Road
Greenville, SC 29615
Phone: 864-627-5337
Fax: 864-627-9301

Spartanburg

Sleep Disorders Center
Spartanburg Regional Medical Center
101 East Wood Street
Spartanburg, SC 29303
Phone: 864-560-6904
Fax: 864-560-7083
E-mail: **SNEWMAN@SRHS.COM**

South Dakota

Rapid City

The Sleep Center
Rapid City Regional Hospital
353 Fairmont Boulevard
PO Box 6000
Rapid City, SD 57709
Phone: 605-719-8037
Fax: 605-719-1924

Sioux Falls

Sleep Disorders Center
Sioux Valley Hospital
1100 South Euclid
Sioux Falls, SD 57117-5039
Phone: 605-333-6302
Fax: 605-333-4402
E-mail: **gravl@siouxvalley.org**

Tennessee

Chattanooga

Parkridge Sleep Disorders Center
Parkridge Medical Center
2333 McCallie Avenue
Plaza II, Suite 300
Chattanooga, TN 37404
Phone: 423-493-6757
Fax: 423-493-6959
E-mail:
**KENDALL.WHITE@HCAHEALTH
CARE.COM**
Web Site:
www.parkridgemedicalcenter.com

Chattanooga

Regional Sleep Center
Memorial Hospital
2525 DeSalles Avenue
Chattanooga, TN 37404
Phone: 423-495-8340
Fax: 423-495-4425
Web Site: **www.memorial.org**

Collierville

BMH Collierville Sleep Disorders
Center
Baptist Memorial Hospital
1500 West Poplar

Collierville, TN 38017
Phone: 901-861-9001
Fax: 901-861-9007
E-mail: **robert.schriner@bmhcc.org**
Web Site: **www.bmhcc.org/services/
hospitals/colliervillesleep.asp**

Cordova

Sleep Labs of Memphis
764 Walnut Knoll Lane
Suite 102
Cordova, TN 38018
Phone: 901-756-4667
Fax: 901-756-4142
E-mail: **sleeplabdirector@cs.com**
Web Site: **midsouthsleep.com**

Hermitage

Summit Center for Sleep Health
Summit Medical Center
5655 Frist Boulevard
Suite 401
Hermitage, TN 37076
Phone: 615-316-3495
Fax: 615-316-3493
E-mail:
Kevin.Justice@HCAhealthcare.com

Knoxville

Sleep Disorders Center
Ft. Sanders Regional Medical Center
1901 West Clinch Avenue
Knoxville, TN 37916
Phone: 865-541-1375
Fax: 865-541-1714

Knoxville

Sleep Disorders Center
St. Mary's Medical Center

900 East Oak Hill Avenue
Knoxville, TN 37917-4556
Phone: 865-545-7529
Fax: 865-545-3115
E-mail: **splenzle@stmaryshealth.com**
Web Site:

Knoxville

The Sleep Center
Baptist Hospital of East Tennessee
PO Box 1788
Knoxville, TN 37901
Phone: 865-632-5627
Fax: 865-549-2176
E-mail: **Skimbro@bhset.org**
Web Site: **www.baptistoneword.org**

Memphis

Sleep Disorders Center
Methodist Hospitals of Memphis
1265 Union Avenue
Memphis, TN 38104
Phone: 901-726-REST
Fax: 901-726-7395

Murfreesboro

Sleep Disorders Center
Middle Tennessee Medical Center
400 North Highland Avenue
Murfreesboro, TN 37130
Phone: 615-849-4811
Fax: 615-849-4833

Nashville

Sleep Disorders Center
Centennial Medical Center
2300 Patterson Street
Nashville, TN 37203
Phone: 615-342-1670

Fax: 615-342-1655
E-mail:
Marcie.Poe@HCAhealthcare.com

Nashville

Sleep Disorders Center
Saint Thomas Hospital
PO Box 380
Nashville, TN 37202
Phone: 615-222-2068
Fax: 615-222-6456
E-mail: **Jburkard@stthomas.org**
Web Site:
www.SAINTTHOMAS.ORG

Nashville

Baptist Sleep Center
Baptist Hospital
2000 Church Street
Nashville, TN 37236
Phone: 615-284-7806
Fax: 615-284-4781
E-mail:
leeann.covington@baptisthospital.com

Oak Ridge

Methodist Sleep Diagnostic Center
Methodist Medical Center
990 Oak Ridge Turnpike
Oak Ridge, TN 37830
Phone: 865-481-1535
Fax: 865-481-1531
E-mail: **kbowling@covhlth.com**
Web Site: **www.mmcoakridge.com**

Texas

Dallas

Sleep Disorders Center for Children
Children's Medical Center of Dallas
1935 Motor Street
Dallas, TX 75235
Phone: 214-456-2793
Fax: 214-456-8740
E-mail:
**JOHERMA@CHILDMED.DALLAS.
TX.US**

Dallas

Sleep Medicine Institute
Presbyterian Hospital of Dallas
8200 Walnut Hill Lane
Dallas, TX 75231
Phone: 214-345-8563
Fax: 214-750-4621
E-mail: **SMAT@sleepmed.com**
Web Site: **www.sleepmed.com**

El Paso

Sleep Disorders Center
Del Sol Medical Center
10301 Gateway West
El Paso, TX 79925
Phone: 915-594-5882
Fax: 915-595-9641
Web Site:
www.delsolmedicalcenter.com

El Paso

Sleep Disorders Center
Providence Memorial Hospital
2001 North Oregon
El Paso, TX 79902
Phone: 915-577-6152

Fax: 915-577-7066
Web Site: **www.sphn.com**

Fort Worth

Sleep Consultants, Inc.
1521 Cooper Street
Fort Worth, TX 76104
Phone: 817-332-7433
Fax: 817-336-2159
E-mail: **info@sleepconsultants.com**
Web Site: **www.sleepconsultants.com**

Houston

Sleep Disorders Center
VA Medical Center and Baylor College
of Medicine
Room 6C344
2002 Holcombe Boulevard
Houston, TX 77030
Phone: 713-794-7563
Fax: 713-794-7558
E-mail: **MAXH@BCM.TMC.EDU**

Houston

Sleep Disorders Center
Hermann Hospital
6411 Fannin Street
Houston, TX 77030
Phone: 713-704-2337
Fax: 713-704-5586
E-mail:
Richard.j.castriotta@uth.tmc.edu
Web Site: **www.salu.net/
hermannsleep/**

Midland

Sleep Center of the Southwest
606 B North Kent Street
Midland, TX 79701

Phone: 915-570-6483
Fax: 915-684-7003
E-mail: **jdavidbray@aol.com**
Web Site: **www.sleepcentersw.com**

Temple

Sleep Disorders Center
Scott and White Clinic
2401 South 31st Street
Temple, TX 76508
Phone: 254-724-2554
Fax: 254-724-2497
E-mail: **fperez-guerra@swmail.sw.org**

Utah

Murray

Intermountain Sleep Disorders Center
of Murray
Cottonwood Hospital
5770 South, 300 East
Murray, UT 84106
Phone: 801-314-2015
Fax: 801-314-2948

Salt Lake City

Intermountain Sleep Disorders Center
LDS Hospital
8th Avenue & C Street
Salt Lake City, UT 84143
Phone: 801-408-3617
Fax: 801-408-5110
E-mail: **ldjwalke@ihc.com**

Salt Lake City

Sleep-Wake Center
University of Utah Hospitals and Clinic
375 Chipeta Way
Suite 200A

Salt Lake City, UT 84108
Phone: 801-581-2016
Fax: 801-587-3349

Vermont

Rutland

The Sleep Center at Rutland Regional
Medical Center
Rutland Regional Medical Center
160 Allen Street
Rutland, VT 05701
Phone: 802-747-3792
Fax: 802-747-6561
E-mail: **sleepctr@rrmc.org**
Web Site: **www.RRMC.ORG**

Virginia

Christiansburg

Sleep Disorders Network
2955 Market Street, Suite B-1
Christiansburg, VA 24073
Phone: 540-382-1165 x102
Fax: 540-382-0989

Norfolk

Sleep Disorders Center for Adults and
Children
Eastern Virginia Medical School
Sentara Norfolk General Hospital
600 Gresham Drive
Norfolk, VA 23507
Phone: 757-668-3322
Fax: 757-668-2628
E-mail: **sleep@evms.edu**
Web Site: **www.evms.edu/sleep/**

Richmond

Sleep Disorders Center
Medical College of Virginia
2529 Professional Road
Richmond, VA 23235
Phone: 804-323-2255
Fax: 804-323-2262
E-mail: RKSOOD@VCU.ORG
Web Site: www.vcu.edu/sleepwell

Richmond

Sleep Disorders Center of Virginia
1800 Glenside Drive, Suite 103
Richmond, VA 23226
Phone: 804-285-0100
Fax: 804-285-2458
E-mail: rparisi@sleepcenter.org
Web Site: www.sleepcenter.org

Roanoke

Carilion Sleep Center
1030 Jefferson Plaza
Suite G100
Roanoke, VA 24016
Phone: 540-985-8526
Fax: 540-985-4963
E-mail: sleep@carilion.com
Web Site: www.carilion.com

Suffolk

Sleep Disorders Center
Obici Hospital
2800 Godwin Boulevard
PO Box 1100
Suffolk, VA 23439-1100
Phone: 757-934-4450
Fax: 757-934-4278
E-mail: lpixley@obici.com
Web Site: www.obici.com

Virginia Beach

Sleep Disorders Center
Sentara Virginia Beach General
Hospital
1060 First Colonial Road
Virginia Beach, VA 23454
Phone: 757-395-8168
Fax: 757-395-6337
E-mail: yxwright@sentara.com

Washington

Auburn

ARMC Sleep Apnea Laboratory*
Auburn Regional Medical Center
Plaza One
202 North Division
Auburn, WA 98001
Phone: 253-804-2809
Fax: 253-333-7599
E-mail: czundel@uhsinc.com
Web Site: auburnregional.com

Lakewood

St. Clare Sleep Related Breathing
Disorders Clinic*
St. Clare Hospital
11315 Bridgeport Way SW
Lakewood, WA 98499
Phone: 253-581-6951
Fax: 253-512-2793

Olympia

Sleep Disorders Center for Southwest
Washington
Providence St. Peter Hospital
413 North Lilly Road
Olympia, WA 98506

Phone: 360-493-7436
Fax: 360-493-4173

Renton

Sleep Center at Valley
Valley Medical Center
400 South 43rd Street
Renton, WA 98055
Phone: 425-656-5340
Fax: 425-793-7382
E-mail: **Barry_Stone@Valleymed.org**
Web Site: **www.valleymed.org**

Richland

Richland Sleep Disorders Center
800 Swift Boulevard
Suite 260
Richland, WA 99352
Phone: 509-946-4632
Fax: 509-946-9791
E-mail: **phamner@owt.com**
Web Site: **www.richsleep.com**

Richland

Columbia Sleep Lab*
780 Swift Boulevard, Suite 130
Richland, WA 99352
Phone: 509-943-6166
Fax: 509-943-8621
E-mail: **Sleepy2400@hotmail.com**

Seattle

Highline Sleep Disorder Center
Highline Community Hospital
14212 Ambaum Boulevard SW
Suite 201
Seattle, WA 98166
Phone: 206-325-7396
Fax: 206-242-2562

Seattle

Sleep Disorders Center, H10-SDC
Virginia Mason Medical Center
925 Seneca Street
Seattle, WA 98111
Phone: 206-625-7180
Fax: 206-341-0447
E-mail: **MSDC@VMMC.ORG**

Seattle

Swedish Sleep Medicine Institute
Swedish Medical Center
801 Broadway
Suite 701
Seattle, WA 98122
Phone: 206-386-2020
Fax: 206-215-3869
E-mail: **bonnie.robertson@swedish.org**

Spokane

Sleep Institute of Spokane
Sacred Heart Doctors Building
105 West Eighth Avenue
Suite 418
Spokane, WA 99204
Phone: 509-455-4895
Fax: 509-343-0155
E-mail: **HURDE@SHMC.ORG**
Web Site: **SHMC.ORG**

Tacoma

MultiCare Sleep Disorders Center
Tacoma General Hospital
PO Box 5299
Tacoma, WA 98405
Phone: 253-403-4554
Fax: 253-403-4553

Walla Walla

Kathryn Severyns Dement Sleep
Disorders Center
St. Mary Medical Center
401 West Poplar
PO Box 1047
Walla Walla, WA 99362
Phone: 509-522-5845
Fax: 509-522-5744
E-mail: **sleepcenter@smmc.com**
Web Site: **www.smmc.com/sleep**

West Virginia

Charleston

Sleep Disorders Center
Charleston Area Medical Center
501 Morris Street
PO Box 1393
Charleston, WV 25325
Phone: 304-388-7507
Fax: 304-388-3373
E-mail: **chuck.menders@camc.org**

Huntington

St. Mary's Regional Sleep Center
St. Mary's Hospital
2900 First Avenue
Huntington, WV 25702
Phone: 304-526-1880
Fax: 304-526-1886
E-mail: **kathy.johnson@st-marys.org**
Web Site: **www.st-marys.org**

Parkersburg

PM Sleep Medicine
3803 Emerson Avenue
PO Box 4179
Parkersburg, WV 26104

Phone: 304-485-5041
Fax: 304-485-5678
Web Site:
www.parkersburg.neurohub.net

South Charleston

Thomas Hospital Sleep Disorder Center
Thomas Memorial Hospital
4605 MacCorkle Avenue SW
South Charleston, WV 25309
Phone: 304-766-3798
Fax: 304-766-3620
E-mail: **priscilla.roberts@thomaswv.org**
Web Site: **www.thomaswv.org**

Wisconsin

Baraboo

St. Clare Hospital Sleep Disorders
Laboratory*
St. Clare Hospital & Health Services
707 14th St.
Baraboo, WI 53913
Phone: 608-355-1752
Fax: 608-355-1742
E-mail: **Lori_Zobel@ssmhc.com**
Web Site: **www.stclare.com**

Chippewa Falls

Marshfield Clinic Sleep Disorders
Center
Chippewa Falls Center
St. Joseph Hospital
2655 County Highway I
Chippewa Falls, WI 54729
Phone: 715-726-4136
Fax: 715-726-4173
E-mail: **Hausmann@mfldclin.edu**

Eau Claire

Luther/Midelfort Sleep Disorders
Center
Luther Hospital/Midelfort Clinic
Mayo Health System
1221 Whipple Street, PO Box 4105
Eau Claire, WI 54702-4105
Phone: 715-838-3886
Fax: 715-838-3266
E-mail:
HRDLICKA.MARY@MAYO.EDU

Green Bay

Sleep Disorders Laboratory*
Bellin Hospital
725 South Webster Avenue
Green Bay, WI 54301
Phone: 920-433-7451
Fax: 920-433-7453
E-mail: **sleeplab@Bellin.org**
Web Site: **www.Bellin.org**

Green Bay

St. Vincent Hospital Sleep Disorders
Center
St. Vincent Hospital
PO Box 13508
Green Bay, WI 54307-3508
Phone: 920-431-3041
Fax: 920-433-8010
E-mail: **mvanlan1@stvgb.org**
Web Site: **www.stvincenthospital.org**

La Crosse

Franciscan Skemp Healthcare Sleep
Laboratory*
Franciscan Skemp Medical Center
700 West Avenue South
La Crosse, WI 54601

Phone: 608-785-0940 x2871
Fax: 608-791-9778
E-mail:
appenzeller.elizabeth@mayo.edu

La Crosse

Wisconsin Sleep Disorders Center
Gundersen Lutheran
1836 South Avenue
La Crosse, WI 54601
Phone: 608-782-7300 x2791
Fax: 608-791-6358
Web Site: **www.gundluth.org**

Madison

Comprehensive Sleep Disorders Center
D6/662 Clinical Science Center
University of Wisconsin Hospitals and
Clinics
600 Highland Avenue
Madison, WI 53792
Phone: 608-263-2387
Fax: 608-265-7229
E-mail:
**SMWEBER2@FACSTAFF.WISC.
EDU**

Madison

Sleep Disorders Center Meriter
Hospital
Meriter Hospital, Inc.
202 South Park Street
Madison, WI 53715
Phone: 608-267-5938
Fax: 608-267-6540
E-mail: **lriley@meriter.com**

Madison

Sleep Disorders Center
St. Marys Hospital Medical Center
707 South Mills Street
Madison, WI 53715
Phone: 608-258-5266
Fax: 608-258-6176
E-mail: **steve_dalebroux@ssmhc.com**

Marshfield

Marshfield Sleep Disorders Center
Marshfield Clinic
1000 North Oak Avenue
Marshfield, WI 54449
Phone: 715-387-5998
Fax: 715-387-5240
E-mail: **Hausmann@mfldclin.edu**
Web Site: **www.marshfieldclinic.org**

Menomonee Falls

Community Memorial Hospital Sleep
Apnea Center
W180 N8085 Town Hall Road
Menomonee Falls, WI 53051
Phone: 262-257-3384
Fax: 262-257-5328
Web Site:
www.communitymemorial.com

Milwaukee

Milwaukee Regional Sleep Disorders
Center
Columbia Hospital
2025 East Newport Avenue
Suite 426Y
Milwaukee, WI 53211
Phone: 414-961-4650
Fax: 414-961-4545

Milwaukee

St. Luke's Sleep Disorders Center
St. Luke's Medical Center
2801 West Kinnickinnic River Parkway
Suite 445
Milwaukee, WI 53215
Phone: 414-649-6573
Fax: 414-649-5875
E-mail: **dave_arnold@aurora.org**

Neenah

Sleep Disorders Center
Theda Clark Medical Center
130 Second Street
Neenah, WI 54946
Phone: 920-729-2901
Fax: 920-729-2902

About the Author:
David O. Volpi M.D.

David O.Volpi M.D., is the Chief of Sleep Disorders at Lenox Hill Hospital's Department of Otolaryngology, Head and Neck Surgery, and has a private Ear, Nose and Throat practice in New York City.

He attended Hahneman Medical College in Philadelphia and completed his post graduate training in General Surgery at the Hospital of The Medical College of Pennsylvania in Philadelphia and a residency in Otolaryngology, Head and Neck Surgery at The New York Medical College Affiliated Hospitals and the New York Eye and Ear Infirmary. He is a Fellow of the American College of Surgeons, as well as a member of the American Academy of Sleep Medicine, the American Medical Association, the Medical Society of the State of New York, the New York County Medical Society, the American Academy of Otolaryngology—Head and Neck Surgery, the American Academy of Facial Plastic and Reconstructive Surgeons and the American Rhinologic Society.

David Volpi is author of several scientific presentations and original papers.

About the Author:
Josh L. Werber M.D.

Josh Werber M.D., is an otolaryngologist who attended New York Medical College and completed his post graduate training in General Surgery at Beth Israel Medical Center and a residency in Otolaryngology/Head and Neck Surgery at the New York Eye and Ear Infirmary in New York City. He also completed a research residency in Normal Tissue Toleranceto Interstitial Radiotherapy at Beth Israel Medical Center and has a private Ear, Nose, and Throat practice in Great Neck, New York.

Josh Werber is author of several scientific presentations and original papers.

Index

0-595-27031-X